Dental Implants

Guest Editor

OLE T. JENSEN, DDS, MS

DENTAL CLINICS OF NORTH AMERICA

www.dental.theclinics.com

October 2011 • Volume 55 • Number 4

SAUNDERS an imprint of ELSEVIER, Inc.

W.B. SAUNDERS COMPANY
A Division of Elsevier Inc.

1600 John F. Kennedy Boulevard ● Suite 1800 ● Philadelphia, Pennsylvania 19103-2899

http://www.dental.theclinics.com

DENTAL CLINICS OF NORTH AMERICA Volume 55, Number 4
October 2011 ISSN 0011-8532, ISBN-978-1-4557-2765-0

Editor: Donald Mumford; D.Mumford@elsevier.com

Dental Clinics of North America (ISSN 0011-8532) is published quarterly by Elsevier Inc., 360 Park Avenue South, New York, NY 10010-1710. Months of issue are January, April, July, and October. Business and Editorial Offices: 1600 John F. Kennedy Boulevard, Suite 1800, Philadelphia, PA 19103-2899. Periodicals postage paid at New York, NY and additional mailing offices. Subscription prices are $240.00 per year (domestic individuals), $420.00 per year (domestic institutions), $113.00 per year (domestic students/residents), $287.00 per year (Canadian individuals), $529.00 per year (Canadian institutions), $347.00 per year (international individuals), $529.00 per year (international institutions), and $170.00 per year (international and Canadian students/residents). International air speed delivery is included in all *Clinics* subscription prices. All prices are subject to change without notice. **POSTMASTER:** Send address changes to *Dental Clinics of North America*, Elsevier Health Sciences Division, Subscription Customer Service, 3251 Riverport Lane, Maryland Heights, MO 63043. **Customer Service (orders, claims, online, change of address): Elsevier Health Sciences Division, Subscription Customer Service, 3251 Riverport Lane, Maryland Heights, MO 63043. Tel: 1-800-654-2452 (U.S. and Canada). Fax: 314-447-8029. E-mail: journalscustomerservice-usa@elsevier.com (for print support); journalsonlinesupport-usa@elsevier.com (for online support).**

Reprints. For copies of 100 or more, of articles in this publication, please contact the Commercial Reprints Department, Elsevier Inc., 360 Park Avenue South, New York, NY 10010-1710. Tel.: 212-633-3812; Fax: 212-462-1935; E-mail: reprints@elsevier.com.

The *Dental Clinics of North America* is covered in *MEDLINE/PubMed (Index Medicus), Current Contents/Clinical Medicine, ISI/BIOMED* and *Clinahl*.

Printed in the United States of America.

Contributors

GUEST EDITOR

OLE T. JENSEN, DDS, MS
Private Practice, Implant Dentistry Associates of Colorado, Greenwood Village, Colorado

AUTHORS

MARCUS ABBOUD, DMD
Associate Professor, Chair of the Department of Prosthodontics and Digital Technology, Stony Brook University School of Dental Medicine, Stony Brook, New York

DEBORA ARMELLINI, DDS, MD
Director of Prosthodontics, ClearChoice, Dental Implant Center–Washington Metro, Vienna, Virginia

EDMOND BEDROSSIAN, DDS, FACD, FACOMS, FAO
Assistant Professor and Director, Implant Training, Department of Oral and Maxillofacial Residency Training Program, Dugoni School of Dentistry, San Francisco, California

MICHAEL S. BLOCK, DMD
The Center for Dental Reconstruction, Metairie, Louisiana

CAESAR C. BUTURA, DDS
Private Practice, ClearChoice Dental Implant Center, Phoenix, Arizona

NARDY CASAP, DMD, MD
Senior Lecturer, Department of Oral and Maxillofacial Surgery, Faculty of Dental Medicine, Hebrew University-Hadassah, Jerusalem, Israel

JARED R. COTTAM, DDS, MS
Private Practice, Burien, Washington

DANIEL F. GALINDO, DDS
Private Practice, ClearChoice Dental Implant Center, Phoenix, Arizona

G.E. GHALI, DDS, MD, FACS
Gamble Professor and Chair, Department of Oral and Maxillofacial Surgery, Head and Neck Surgery, Louisiana State University Health Sciences Center Shreveport, Shreveport, Louisiana

STUART GRAVES, DDS, MS
Oral Surgeon, Private Practice, Burke, Virginia

BEN JAVID, DDS
Prosthodontist, Private Practice, Rockville, Maryland

OLE T. JENSEN, DDS, MS
Private Practice, Implant Dentistry Associates of Colorado, Greenwood Village, Colorado

D. DAVID KIM, DMD, MD, FACS
Associate Professor, Department of Oral and Maxillofacial Surgery, Head and Neck Surgery, Louisiana State University Health Sciences Center Shreveport, Shreveport, Louisiana

ZVI LASTER, DMD
Head, Oral and Maxillofacial Surgery Department, The Baruch Padeh Medical Center, Poriya, Tiberias, Israel

DANIEL LESMES, DMD
Formerly, Chief Resident, Oral and Maxillofacial Surgery Department, The Baruch Padeh Medical Center, Poriya, Tiberias; Currently, Consultant, Oral and Maxillofacial Unit, The Rivka Ziv Medical Center, Safed, Israel

PATRICK J. LOUIS, DDS, MD
Professor and Residency Program Director, Oral and Maxillofacial Surgery, School of Dentistry, University of Alabama at Birmingham, Birmingham, Alabama

BRIAN A. MAHLER, DDS
Private Practice Limited to Prosthodontics, Fairfax, Virginia

ROBERT E. MARX, DDS
Professor of Surgery and Chief, Division of Oral and Maxillofacial Surgery, University of Miami, Miller School of Medicine, Miami, Florida

CRAIG M. MISCH, DDS, MDS
Private Practice, Oral and Maxillofacial Surgery and Prosthodontics, Sarasota, Florida; Clinical Associate Professor, Department of Implant Dentistry, New York University College of Dentistry, New York, New York

GARY ORENTLICHER, DMD
Private Practice, New York Oral, Maxillofacial, and Implant Surgery, Scarsdale; Section Chief, Oral and Maxillofacial Surgery, White Plains Hospital, White Plains, New York

JASON L. RINGEMAN, DDS, MD
Fellow, Tissue Engineering Institute of Colorado, Greenwood Village, Colorado

DOUGLAS P. SINN, DDS, FACD
Clinical Professor and Past Chairman, Division of Oral and Maxillofacial Surgery, Department of Surgery, UT Southwestern Medical School at Dallas, Dallas, Texas

DANIEL B. SPAGNOLI, MS, PhD, DDS
University Oral and Maxillofacial Surgery, Charlotte, North Carolina

ALLISON K. VEST, MBBS, MS, CCA
Anaplastologist, Medical Arts Prosthetics, LLC, Dallas, Texas

Contents

> The use of osseointegrated dental implants has gained momentum, mainly in the last 20 years. Research and development in the field of implantology are constantly focusing on implant redesign to continue to try and improve implant success. The current aim of implant design is to address situations prone to failure, such as cases of low bone quality or cases of concomitant systemic diseases that compromise healing.

> This article discusses the management of the facial gingival margin before and after tooth removal. Important factors including diagnostic assessment, wound healing, bone resorption and remodeling, gingival thickness, and gingival margin are reviewed, and key procedures suggested. Gingival thickness can have a major influence on the maintenance of the facial gingival margin over the longer term.

> Many bone grafting techniques have been used to reconstruct the partially dentate and edentulous mandible. This article discusses the various bone grafting techniques to reconstruct mandibular defects. Also included are issues such as whether autogenous bone is necessary for reconstruction of the mandibular ridge and the importance of membranes.

> Reconstruction of the atrophic maxilla for dental implant placement has many unique considerations. There are several methods available to augment the atrophic maxilla. Of these, autogenous bone grafting offers a well-proven predictable method for ridge augmentation and defect repair for dental implant placement. There are several advantages of using autogenous bone grafts. This article primarily focuses on the use of autogenous onlay bone grafts to reconstruct the atrophic maxilla.

> New three-dimensional diagnostic and treatment planning technologies in implant dentistry have expanded on concepts of a team approach to the

planning and placement of dental implants. The accurate and predictable placement of implants according to a computer-generated virtual treatment plan is now a reality, taking the virtual plan from the computer to the patient clinically. Recent advances in three-dimensional imaging in dentistry, in combination with the introduction of third-party proprietary implant planning software and associated surgical instrumentation, have revolutionized dental implant diagnosis and treatment and created an interdisciplinary environment in which communication leads to better patient care and outcomes.

The use of "anteriorly or posteriorly" tilted implants in a graftless approach for immediate loading the edentulous maxillae has been well documented in the literature. This treatment concept allows for rehabilitation of the edentulous maxillae with a fixed prosthesis. The purpose of this article is to describe criteria for the use of the zygomatic implant, including the expanded use of the zygoma implant in cases where failure of one of the anterior or posterior tilted implants has occurred in the All-on-Four treatment concept. Zygomatic implant placement becomes a "rescue procedure", which allows for continuity of care without resorting to a removable denture.

The maxilla is a challenging area for dental implant restoration. Encroachment of anatomic structures such as the sinus and nasal floor make vertical placement difficult. Implants placed at an angle may be used to avoid these anatomic structures or eliminate the need for a bone grafting procedure. The question occasionally arises about the possible detrimental effects of placing implants at an angle. This article reviews relevant literature, presents two case reports on maxillary angled implants and presents 3 years of data on 276 All-on-Four restorations.

Immediate function with Brånemark implants is well established for the mandible. This article describes a series of 857 implants placed consecutively in which very few implants failed or lost bone despite the dynamic healing conditions of simultaneous dental extractions and bone leveling. Though these findings are relatively early, 3 years or fewer, it appears that the immediate function All-on-Four procedure can be done with a high degree of confidence for the mandible—putting into question the need for additional implants.

THE CLINICS ARE NOW AVAILABLE ONLINE!

Access your subscription at:
www.theclinics.com

Preface

Oral and Craniofacial Implant Reconstruction as Foundation for Restorative Dentistry

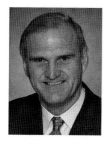

Ole T. Jensen, DDS, MS
Guest Editor

Dental implant reconstruction, including craniofacial reconstruction, is an evolving art and science: an art, because there is still no absolute prescription for any given situation; a science, because after placement of millions of dental implants worldwide, scientific knowledge is still expanding exponentially.

To contemplate repair of a defect is to seek enlightenment from master clinicians experienced in settings as disparate as gingival esthetics and cancer reconstruction. But there is still controversy as to which therapy to use in any given situation. Optimally, tissue engineering will enable regeneration of all regional tissues, obtaining form and function not based on prosthetic elements. At present though, the titanium bone screw, in use these past four decades, remains the mainstay of most all oral and craniofacial reconstructive efforts, and therefore, a foundation for restorative dentistry.

This issue *of Dental Clinics of North America* discusses current thinking of the most challenging settings for the reconstructive surgeon and therefore the restorative dentist, from the single missing tooth in the esthetic zone to complete loss of craniofacial structure. Hopefully, this review will update the restorative dentist to enable better understanding of the broad range of methods that have lately become "standardized," including the fibula flap, BMP-2 repair, all on four immediate function, and computer guidance.

Ole T. Jensen, DDS, MS
Implant Dentistry Associates of Colorado
8200 East Belleview Avenue
Suite 520E
Greenwood Village, CO 80111, USA

E-mail address:
ole.jensen@clearchoice.com

Dent Clin N Am 55 (2011) ix
doi:10.1016/j.cden.2011.08.001
dental.theclinics.com

Innovations in Dental Implant Design for Current Therapy

Daniel Lesmes, DMD[a,b], Zvi Laster, DMD[b],*

KEYWORDS

- Dental implant design • Systemic disease
- Osseointegrated dental implants

Since Branemark coined the term osseointegration following his 1952 accidental discovery, the use of osseointegrated dental implants has gained momentum, mainly in the last 20 years.[1,2] Dental implants are now the state of the art for dental restorative therapy. Yet, research and development in the field of implantology are constantly focusing on implant redesign (eg, topography, implant surface, macro-design) to continue to try and improve implant success. The current aim of implant design is to address situations prone to failure, such as cases of low bone quality or cases of concomitant systemic diseases that compromise healing such as diabetes mellitus.

As opposed to other implants used throughout the human body, the dental implant presents with a unique dual complexity. The implant must engage bone to become osseointegrated but also presents outside the body in the oral cavity connected to a prosthetic tooth.

Today, there are over 1300 dental implant types, each with differing properties: size, shape, and surface. Emerging new developments are based mainly on modification of either chemical or mechanical properties of an implant. Thus, it is expected to improve host tissue response and accelerate the healing process.

Clinical findings suggest that these changes, particularly in implant surface design, have contributed immensely to dental implant success.[3,4] Nevertheless, implant macrotopography also has made a contribution.[5]

The aim of this article is to present a comprehensive review of current innovations in dental implant design and discuss variations in bone stock that may impact a clinician's implant selection.

This article was previously published in the May 2011 issue of *Oral and Maxillofacial Surgery Clinics of North America*.
[a] Oral and Maxillofacial Unit, Rivka Ziv Medical Center, Safed 13000, Israel
[b] Oral and Maxillofacial Surgery Department, The Baruch Padeh Medical Center, Poriya, Tiberias 15208, Israel
* Corresponding author.
E-mail address: zvi@lasters.co.il

Dent Clin N Am 55 (2011) 649–661
doi:10.1016/j.cden.2011.07.004
0011-8532/11/$ – see front matter © 2011 Elsevier Inc. All rights reserved.

DENTAL IMPLANT SURFACE MICRO-TOPOGRAPHY

Since the mid-1980s, a rationale for roughened titanium surfaces compared with turned titanium (smooth) has been formalized.[3,6,7]

Roughened titanium surfaces appear to provide micromechanical locking at the micrometric scale and at the same time enhance superior osseointegration by absorption of ions and proteins after implant tissue contact has been achieved, while smooth surfaces do not.[8] Moreover, implant design and surface technology may have an influence on marginal bone response during immediate functional loading.

Several experimental investigations have demonstrated that bone response is influenced by implant surface. Relatively smooth (S(a) <0.5 µm) and minimally rough (S(a) 0.5–1 µm) surfaces showed less strong bone responses than rougher surfaces.[9] However, this microarchitecture does not substantially contribute to primary implant stability.

Immediate loading is among the most innovative techniques used in implant therapy today. The biomechanical outcome of various designs and surfaces that claim to shorten implant treatment is the focus of intense academic debate. The biomechanical outcome of various designs and surfaces claims to shorten implant treatment time.[10] One animal study showed that the highest mean removal torque values were recorded with a bone screw with a wide thread profile (titanium plasma spray coating) at 24.4 Newton per centimeters (NCm)/mm followed by thread profiles that were sandblated and acid-etched at 22.3 NCm/mm. A low thread profile (anodic oxidized surface) was next at 18.7 NCm/mm. The lowest score was obtained by low thread (double-etched and machined surface) at 12.0 NCm/mm. The authors concluded that immediate loading was possible with various designs and surfaces, but when high primary stability was needed, an aggressive thread profile was best.

A retrospective human study concluded that there was no impact of design or surface treatment on implant survival in the completely edentulous mandible where most immediate load experience has been reported clinically.[11] Bone preservation in immediately loaded implants in the mandible appears to be influenced by implant design and was significantly better on surface-modified AstraTech implants (Astra Tech AB, Mölndal, Sweden) compared with machined Branemark implants (Branemark Implant System, Nobel Biocare, Zürich-Flughafen, Switzerland). In the mandible, a microthread design of the implant collar did not seem to improve bone preservation.

One thing to consider in implant design is bone quality. If the mandible is taken as a baseline example, according to Lekholm and Zarb, there may be 4 different types of bone present, from high cortical content (type 1) to poorly mineralized, even osteoporotic (type 4).[12–14]

Fig. 1 shows a schematic of these proposed bone quality differences. Although the relationship of the drill preparation to the diameter of the implant is very important, implant insertion may be optimized by using bone screw designs that are specifically made to address bone type. Examples of 4 different implants are illustrated in **Fig. 1**, including their use in angulated placement strategies. Suggested by the schematic is that the surgeon may make implant selection based on clinical criteria of operative bone density.

Despite the varied implant designs available for use in different bone density situations, the surgeon can most often adapt techniques to control insertion torque and therefore primary stability no matter what implant type is used. For example, by using a 1° to 2° tapered implant, placed with a straight, often stepped-down bur, implants can gain fixation in both hard and soft bone provided the implant has self-tapping threads for hard bone. By underpreparation, poorly mineralized bone can still secure implant fixation.

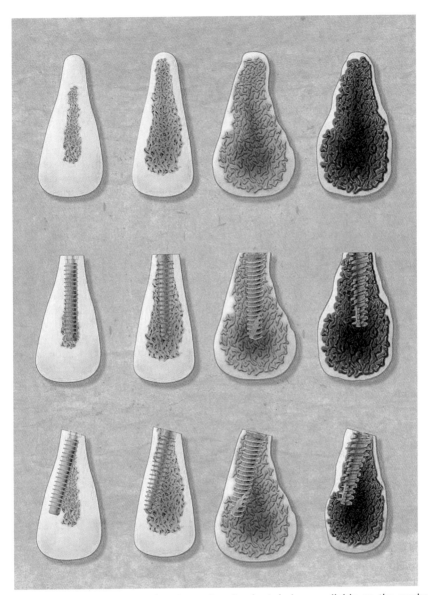

Fig. 1. This rendering suggests that the various implant designs available on the market-place do not always work in all types of bone, even though by altering surgical techniques surgeons are able to make almost any type of implant work no matter the osseous finding. In general, a finer thread pitch is more suitable for dense bone usually placed after screw tapping. Softer bone situations are accommodated best by the use of aggressive threaded implants with a mild taper, which are more likely to gain adequate insertion torque for immediate function.

By tapping or the use of hard bone drills (overpreparation) in type 1 bone, most implant designs can still be used to gain fixation by modifying the surgical technique.

In the special situation of use of an implant in osteoid, such as found in newly forming bone in large BMP-2 grafts, an aggressive implant design is better, as the cortex may be absent and mineralization content is often much less than 15%.

An example of the use of an aggressive threaded implant used in an extraction site associated with soft bone for immediate temporization is seen in **Figs. 2–8**.

IMPLANT SURFACE CHEMICAL PROPERTIES

The implant surface energy and wetting capability influence the ability to absorb biomolecules, mainly plasma proteins, thus affecting the first phase of osseointegration.

Rough-surfaced implants are known to have hydrophobic properties. When in contact with body fluids, these surfaces show hydrophilic traits, a phenomenon of air microbubble entrapment at the dry surface.[13,14]

Implant surface properties influence resonance frequency analysis measurements of implant stability. Surface chemistry-modified titanium implants showed higher mean implant stability values than did topographically changed implants. In particular, cation (magnesium)-incorporated micropatterns in magnesium incorporated implants may play a primary role in implant stability.[15]

Implants with nanometer-scale surface topography (NanoTite BIOMET 3i, Palm Beach Gardens, FL, USA) were created by discrete crystalline depositions (DCDs) of calcium phosphate nanocrystals onto a dual acid-etched (DAE) surface. These implants show enhanced early fixation in preclinical studies when compared with DAE-surfaced implants. A clinical study showed a cumulative survival rate of 94.9% after 1 year. Relative to other prospective, multicenter studies of immediately loaded implants with various surface enhancements, NanoTite implants perform comparatively well when immediately provisionalized with single-tooth and fixed restorations.[16]

Surface chemistry also appears to play a significant role in cell response to sandblasted and acid-etched surfaces in the presence of titanium hydride TiH[(2)], which may promote attachment, proliferation, and differentiation of preosteoblasts.[17]

BIOACTIVE COATING AND PROCESSING

There is a great demand for dental implant surfaces to accelerate the process of peri-implant bone generation to reduce healing time and enable early loading.

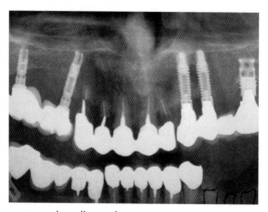

Fig. 2. Preoperative panoramic radiograph.

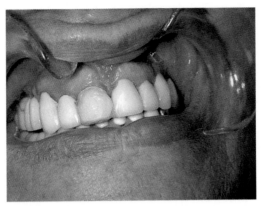

Fig. 3. Preoperative intraoral view.

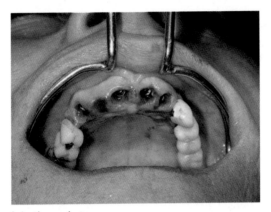

Fig. 4. Implants sunk in the sockets.

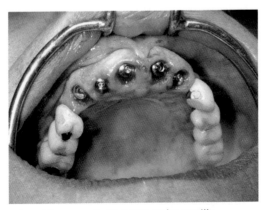

Fig. 5. Healing caps placed temporarily to support the papilla.

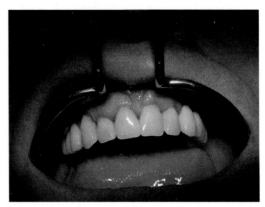

Fig. 6. Temporary reinforced bridge placed after 2 days.

To improve tissue integration, the neck region of dental implants was coated with biodegradable polymer poly (L-lactide) incorporating tetracycline, ibuprofen, and the combination of both drugs. Results showed a continuous release of the embedded drugs in relevant dosages over a period of 6 months. In contrast to high tetracycline concentrations, high ibuprofen concentrations resulted in a decreased metabolic activity.[18]

For orthopedic and dental implants, the ultimate goal is to obtain life-long anchoring of the implant to native bone. To this end, nanoscale calcium phosphate (CaP) and collagen-CaP (col-CaP) composite coatings have been deposited. In vitro cell culture experiments showed that electrosprayed CaP and col-CaP composite coatings enhanced osteoblast differentiation, leading to improved mineral deposition. This effect was most pronounced upon codeposition of collagen with CaP.[19]

A modified titanium surface, anodized after being discharged in electrolytes, provides antibacterial activity against oral bacteria and provides for osteoconductivity.[20] To study this, titanium plates are anodized in various electrolytes with or without chloride. Then, the survival of *Streptococcus mutans* plated on the surface of each

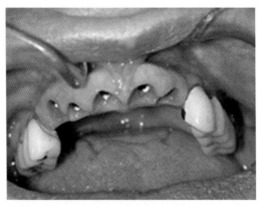

Fig. 7. Temporary reinforced bridge is removed for impression.

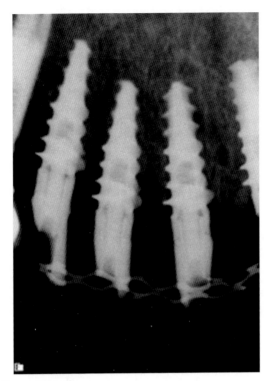

Fig. 8. Postoperative radiograph.

specimen was evaluated. Chloride solutions efficiently killed adherent *S mutans*, whereas the presence of hydrophilicity alone did not demonstrate antibacterial activity. Therefore, this method of anodizing the titanium surface in a chloride solution may provide a novel strategy for use in orthopedic or dental implant systems.[20]

DENTAL IMPLANT GROSS TOPOGRAPHY

Implant geometry and collar macrostructure and microstructure affect crestal bone height, soft tissue mobility values, and attachment levels. In a paper comparing rough with smooth-collared implants and at the same time investigating stepped versus straight-collared implants, there were statistically significant differences in attachment levels. Implants with straight collars had less bone loss at the 5-year interval than implants with stepped collars. Bone level changes were greater when the implant was placed further subcrestal.[21]

To evaluate the effect of implant threads, two models were created by Assuncao and colleagues: a model in which the implant threads were accurately simulated, and a model in which implants with a smooth surface (press-fit implant) were used. The threaded model showed higher maximum stress values (1.45 MPa) than the press-fit model (1.2 MPa). When in cortical bone, stress values differed by about 36%, whereas in trabecular bone, the stress distribution and stress values were similar. Considering implant and cortical bone analysis, remarkable differences in stress values were found between the models. Although the models showed different absolute stress values, the stress distribution was similar.[22]

Whereas most endosseous dental implants have threaded screw-form geometries, press-fit implants integrate via 3-dimensional bone ingrowth. These two classes of implants are well suited for different site conditions, and, when used appropriately, can provide optimal and minimally invasive treatment protocols. Threaded implants are more appropriate for immediate placement and immediate loading, while press-fit implants may perform well in resorbed posterior sites, including maxillary sites with as little as 3 mm of subantral bone. Generally, threaded screw implants perform best in long lengths (with a defined intrabony length above 8 mm) and denser bone, while press-fit sintered porous-surfaced implants perform optimally at short lengths (defined intrabony length of 5 mm or less) and in primarily cancellous bone.[5]

Different implant configurations influence the amount of buccal/palatal bone loss that occurs during the first phases of healing following installation into extraction sockets.[23] Sanz and colleagues conducted a prospective, randomized-controlled parallel-group multicenter study in which either a cylindrical or a tapered implant was placed into anterior maxillary extraction sockets. The study demonstrated that the removal of a single tooth and the immediate placement of an implant resulted in marked alteration of the dimension of the buccal ridge. The horizontal and vertical gaps between the implant and the bone walls were studied. Although the dimensional changes were not significantly different between the 2-implant configurations, both the horizontal and the vertical gap changes were greater in the cylindrical implant group than in the tapered implant group.

Factors such as thread pitch, thread geometry, helix angle, thread depth and width, as well as the implant crestal module may affect implant stability. A decreased thread pitch may positively influence implant stability. Excess helix angles in spite of a faster insertion may jeopardize the ability of implants to sustain axial load. Deeper threads seem to have an important effect on the stabilization in poorer bone quality but are difficult to use in dense bone. The addition of threads or microthreads up to the crestal module of an implant might provide a potential positive contribution on bone-to-implant contact as well as on the preservation of marginal bone; nonetheless this remains to be determined.[24]

ZIRCONIA IMPLANTS

Ceramics have been used in dentistry and medicine for many years. Today, one of the most popular ceramics is zirconia because of its outstanding mechanical properties, which makes it suitable for many indications formerly reserved for metals. Currently, zirconia is widely used in the biomedical arena as a material for prosthetic devices because of its good mechanical and chemical properties. Largely employed for total hip replacement, zirconia ceramics (ZrO(2)) are becoming prevalent in dentistry and dental implantology, including the manufacture of implants completely made of zirconia (Ceraroot Incorporated, Barcelona, Spain).

The successful use of zirconia ceramics in orthopedic surgery led to a demand for dental zirconium-based implant systems.

Zirconia oral implants are a new topic in implant dentistry, and recently, some articles in the dental literature have suggested the possible use of zirconia implants for tooth replacement as shown in **Fig. 9**. So far, no controlled clinical studies in people regarding clinical outcomes or osseointegration could be identified. Clinical data are still restricted to case studies, case series, and animal studies.[25–31] Nevertheless, the data available on the biologic and biomechanical behavior are of importance to understand and perhaps may enhance the future of implant dentistry.

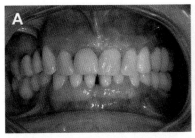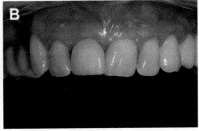

Fig. 9. (*A, B*) The right central incisor following restoration with the zirconium implant with perfect color match of marginal gingival.

Orthopedic and dental implant biomaterials are expected to be in contact with living tissues for a long period of time, and long-term toxicity must be carefully evaluated. Zirconia biomaterials are suitable for biomedical applications and have no carcinogenic effect. For example, Maccauro and colleagues[31] report the development of a new zirconia material with interesting properties, both from a mechanical and a biocompatibility point of view. Further studies are needed to determine its suitability as a candidate biomaterial for orthopedic implants and dental devices.

Osseointegration is crucial for long-term success of dental implants and depends on the tissue reaction at the tissue–implant interface. Mechanical properties and biocompatibility make zirconia a suitable material for dental implants, although surface processing is still problematic. Zirconia implants with modified surfaces result in an osseointegration, which is comparable with that of titanium implants, both at the macro and at the ultrastructural level.[32–35] Significant modifications, such as macroretentions, seem to indicate that primary stability and excellent osseointegration of immediate root analog zirconia implants can be achieved, while preventing unaesthetic bone resorption (see **Fig. 9**; **Figs. 10–14**).[14] Therefore, zirconia implants may have the potential to become an alternative to titanium implants but cannot currently be recommended for routine clinical use, as no long-term clinical data are available.

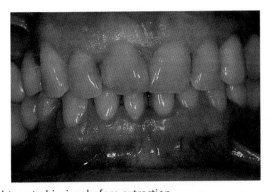

Fig. 10. Failed right central incisor before extraction.

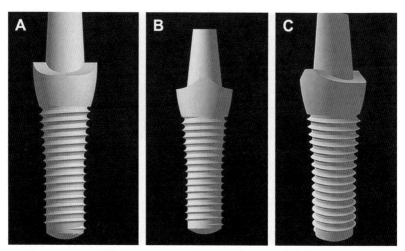

Fig. 11. (A–C) One-piece zirconium implant with scalloped abutment platform (CeraRoot Incorporated, Barcelona, Spain).

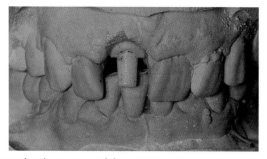

Fig. 12. Abutment analog in stone model.

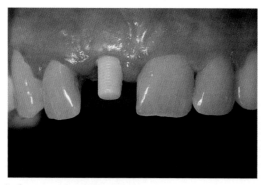

Fig. 13. Abutment before crown cementation.

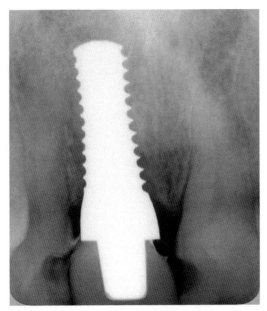

Fig. 14. The well osseointegrated zirconium implant 1 year after restoration.

REFERENCES

1. Branemark PI. Osseointegration and its experimental background. J Prosthet Dent 1983;50(3):399–410.
2. Albrektsson T, Brånemark PI, Hansson HA, et al. Osseointegrated titanium implants. Requirements for ensuring a long-lasting, direct bone-to-implant anchorage in man. Acta Orthop Scand 1981;52(2):155–70.
3. Trisi P, Lazzara R, Rao W, et al. Bone implant contact on machined and dual acid-etched surfaces after 2 months of healing in the human maxilla. J Periodontol 2003;74(7):945–56.
4. Buser D, Schenk RK, Steinemann S, et al. Influence of surface characteristics on bone integration of titanium implants. A histomorphometric study in miniature pigs. J Biomed Mater Res 1991;25(7):889–902.
5. Deporter D. Dental implant design and optimal treatment outcomes. Int J Periodontics Restorative Dent 2009;29(6):625–33.
6. Albrektsson T, Wennerberg A. Oral implant surfaces: part 1—review focusing on topographic and chemical properties of different surfaces and in vivo responses to them. Int J Prosthodont 2004;17(5):536–43.
7. Khang W, Feldman S, Hawley CE, et al. A multicenter study comparing dual acid-etched and machined-surfaced implants in various bone qualities. J Periodontol 2001;72(10):1384–90.
8. Le Guehennec L, Soueidan A, Layrolle P, et al. Surface treatments of titanium dental implants for rapid osseointegration. Dent Mater 2007;23(7):844–54.
9. Wennerberg A, Albrektsson T. Effects of titanium surface topography on bone integration: a systematic review. Clin Oral Implants Res 2009;20(Suppl 4):172–84.
10. Neugebauer J, Weinländer M, Lekovic V, et al. Mechanical stability of immediately loaded implants with various surfaces and designs: a pilot study in dogs. Int J Oral Maxillofac Implants 2009;24(6):1083–92.

11. Van de Velde T, Collaert B, Sennerby L, et al. Effect of implant design on preservation of marginal bone in the mandible. Clin Implant Dent Relat Res 2010;12(2): 134–41.

12. Sul YT, Johansson C, Wennerberg A, et al. Optimum surface properties of oxidized implants for reinforcement of osseointegration: surface chemistry, oxide thickness, porosity, roughness, and crystal structure. Int J Oral Maxillofac Implants 2005;20(3):349–59.

13. Sul YT, Jönsson J, Yoon GS, et al. Resonance frequency measurements in vivo and related surface properties of magnesium-incorporated, micropatterned and magnesium-incorporated TiUnite, Osseotite, SLA and TiOblast implants. Clin Oral Implants Res 2009;20(10):1146–55.

14. Lekholm U, Zarb GA. Patient selection. In: Branenmark PI, Zarb GA, Albrektsson T, editors. Tissue-integrated prostheses: osseointegration in clinical dentistry. Chicago: Quintessence; 1985. p. 199–209.

15. Ostman PO, Hupalo M, del Castillo R, et al. Immediate provisionalization of Nano-Tite implants in support of single-tooth and unilateral restorations: one-year interim report of a prospective, multicenter study. Clin Implant Dent Relat Res 2010;12(Suppl 1):e47–55.

16. Zhang F, Yang GL, He FM, et al. Cell response of titanium implant with a roughened surface containing titanium hydride: an in vitro study. J Oral Maxillofac Surg 2010;68(5):1131–9.

17. Wolf J, Sternberg K, Behrend D, et al. Drug release of coated dental implant neck region to improve tissue integration. Biomed Tech (Berl) 2009;54(4):219–27.

18. de Jonge LT, Leeuwenburgh SC, van den Beucken JJ, et al. The osteogenic effect of electrosprayed nanoscale collagen/calcium phosphate coatings on titanium. Biomaterials 2010;31(9):2461–9.

19. Deng JY, Arimoto T, Shibata Y, et al. Role of chloride formed on anodized titanium surfaces against an oral microorganism. J Biomater Appl 2010;25(2):179–89.

20. Stein AE, McGlmphy EA, Johnston WM, et al. Effects of implant design and surface roughness on crestal bone and soft tissue levels in the esthetic zone. Int J Oral Maxillofac Implants 2009;24(5):910–9.

21. Assuncao WG, Gomes EA, Barão VA, et al. Stress analysis in simulation models with or without implant threads representation. Int J Oral Maxillofac Implants 2009;24(6):1040–4.

22. Vignoletti F, Johansson C, Albrektsson T, et al. Early healing of implants placed into fresh extraction sockets: an experimental study in the beagle dog. De novo bone formation. J Clin Periodontol 2009;36(3):265–77.

23. Abuhussein H, Pagni G, Rebaudi A, et al. The effect of thread pattern upon implant osseointegration. Clin Oral Implants Res 2010;21(2):129–36.

24. Kohal RJ, Wolkewitz M, Hinze M, et al. Biomechanical and histological behavior of zirconia implants: an experiment in the rat. Clin Oral Implants Res 2009;20(4): 333–9.

25. Wenz HJ, Bartsch J, Wolfart S, et al. Osseointegration and clinical success of zirconia dental implants: a systematic review. Int J Prosthodont 2008;21(1): 27–36.

26. Stubinger S, Homann F, Etter C, et al. Effect of Er:YAG, CO(2) and diode laser irradiation on surface properties of zirconia endosseous dental implants. Lasers Surg Med 2008;40(3):223–8.

27. Rocchietta I, Fontana F, Addis A, et al. Surface-modified zirconia implants: tissue response in rabbits. Clin Oral Implants Res 2009;20(8):844–50.

28. Lee J, Sieweke JH, Rodriguez NA, et al. Evaluation of nano-technology-modified zirconia oral implants: a study in rabbits. J Clin Periodontol 2009;36(7):610–7.

29. Langhoff JD, Voelter K, Scharnweber D, et al. Comparison of chemically and pharmaceutically modified titanium and zirconia implant surfaces in dentistry: a study in sheep. Int J Oral Maxillofac Surg 2008;37(12):1125–32.

30. Gahlert M, Röhling S, Wieland M, et al. Osseointegration of zirconia and titanium dental implants: a histological and histomorphometrical study in the maxilla of pigs. Clin Oral Implants Res 2009;20(11):1247–53.

31. Maccauro G, Bianchino G, Sangiorgi S, et al. Development of a new zirconia-toughened alumina: promising mechanical properties and absence of in vitro carcinogenicity. Int J Immunopathol Pharmacol 2009;22(3):773–9.

32. Depprich R, Zipprich H, Ommerborn M, et al. Osseointegration of zirconia implants compared with titanium: an in vivo study. Head Face Med 2008;4:30.

33. Depprich R, Zipprich H, Ommerborn M, et al. Osseointegration of zirconia implants: an SEM observation of the bone–implant interface. Head Face Med 2008;4:25.

34. Depprich R, Ommerborn M, Zipprich H, et al. Behavior of osteoblastic cells cultured on titanium and structured zirconia surfaces. Head Face Med 2008;4:29.

35. Pirker W, Kocher A. Immediate, nonsubmerged, root analogue zirconia implants placed into single-rooted extraction sockets: 2-year follow-up of a clinical study. Int J Oral Maxillofac Surg 2009;38(11):1127–32.

Management of the Facial Gingival Margin

Michael S. Block, DMD

KEYWORDS

- Facial gingival margin • Tooth removal • Bone resorption
- Gingival thickness

DIAGNOSTIC ASSESSMENT

Clinical observations are used to evaluate a patient's facial appearance.[1] For the esthetic implant restoration, 4 critical areas to document in the initial evaluation include: (1) the smile line and incisor show at rest; (2) the length of the incisor that sets the ideal location of the facial gingival margin; (3) the bone morphology under the gingiva; and (4) the thickness of the patient's gingiva.

The smile line sets the vertical location of the incisor edge of the maxillary central incisors. Typically the exposure of the central incisor at rest with the lips relaxed and apart is 2 to 4 mm, depending on the patient's age and gender. As the patient ages he or she tends to show less maxillary tooth at rest. The clinician notes the location of the incisor edge and then may need to fabricate a setup with the ideal location of the incisor edge. This is one of the critical factors when determining the ultimate position of the facial gingival margin.[2,3]

The length of the central incisor sets the ideal location of the gingival margin. The central incisor is typically 10.5 to 11.0 mm in length. Once the planned, ideal incisor edge position is known, then the ideal location of the facial gingival margin can be established by using the standard 11-mm tall central incisor to apically identify the ideal position of the facial gingival margin.[4–7]

Diagnostic assessment must also include the quantity and shape of the bone at the crest of the planned implant site. The horizontal projection of the crestal bone and its height will set the stage for the location of the facial gingival margin of the planned implant restoration. If the bone is not sufficient then the facial gingival margin may be apical to ideal, and also may not project forward to simulate root form eminence of a natural tooth in the esthetic zone.

This article was previously published in the May 2011 issue of *Oral and Maxillofacial Surgery Clinics of North America*.

The Center for Dental Reconstruction, 111 Veterans Memorial Boulevard, Suite 112, Metairie, LA 70005, USA

E-mail address: drblock@crdnola.com

Dent Clin N Am 55 (2011) 663–671
doi:10.1016/j.cden.2011.07.005
0011-8532/11/$ – see front matter

dental.theclinics.com

The thickness of the gingiva will be predictive concerning the long-term vertical movement or lack of movement of the facial gingival margin. In the patient with thin gingiva, underlying bone remodeling and apical resorption of the crestal bone will lead to gingival recession. The patient with thick gingiva will have less apical movement over time as bone remodels.[8-10] It may be important to convert the thin gingiva over an implant site to thick gingiva to slow the process of gingival recession as bone continues to remodel over time.[9,10]

The critical points mentioned can be combined with 4 additional basic observations of wound healing. These 4 wound healing keys will affect the clinical choices made by the surgeon and restorative dentist as concerns which adjunctive therapies are used when restoring a missing tooth in the esthetic zone of the maxilla.

Keys to remember:

1. Thin bone resorbs over time. The labial bone over an anterior maxillary tooth is usually less than 1.5 mm thick, and may be less than 1.0 mm thick. There is evidence that the natural progression of labial bone thickness is for it to decrease up to 1.0 mm after the implant is placed. If thin bone resorbs then the implant's surface may become exposed to the soft tissues, with subsequent recession and loss of esthetic appearance.[11]
2. Thin gingiva recedes over time. If the final crown is placed on an anterior maxillary implant with facial gingival margin perfectly located, then subsequent gingival recession will adversely affect the appearance of the patient. In the patient with thick gingiva bone, remodeling apically will result in pocket formation with minimal recession. However, in the patient with thin gingiva bone, remodeling in the apical direction will result in gingival recession and lengthening of the tooth with a poor esthetic result.[12]
3. Allograft particles are resorbed as bone formation occurs, with decrease of the graft volume. Bone resorption of grafts can result in flattening of the crest and an unnatural appearance with loss of the natural root eminence. This point is important to consider when immediately placing an implant into an extraction site, with a gap between the labial surface of the implant and a thin labial cortical plate of bone. If allograft is used and the labial bone resorbs, which is expected, combined with allograft volume thinning, then the ultimate appearance of the site is flat. The use of a relatively nonresorbable material may prevent the development of a flat ridge.
4. The remodeling of bone through healing of a bone defect follows a defined course, which can be minimally affected by grafting. When the clinician recognizes this process then different approaches to the site can be utilized to "mask" bone remodeling and thinning.

EVIDENCE TO SUPPORT THE AFOREMENTIONED KEYS

Bone remodeling occurs in the crestal region after tooth removal. Block and Kent[13] demonstrated in a dog model that bone will remodel and thin in the crestal area when no graft material is placed in a fresh extraction socket. When particulate hydroxyapatite was placed into the fresh extraction sites, ridge form was maintained. However, histologic evidence showed that the bone remodeled in a very similar pattern, mimicking the normal extraction site healing. Bone was not preserved by the grafting process, only the presence of the nonresorbable material maintained ridge form.[13] This result supports the use of a sintered bovine material, which is relatively nonresorbable as a graft, between the labial surface of an implant and intact thin labial bone, anticipating bone resorption but maintaining the appearance of root form eminence by the presence of the sintered xenograft.

Bone remodeling is a natural process after surgical procedures as well as after tooth removal and implant placement. Cardaropoli and colleagues[11] showed that from the time of abutment connection, a mean loss of bone height at the facial and lingual aspect of the implant amounted to 0.7 to 1.3 mm (P<.05), whereas no significant change was noted at proximal sites. A mean reduction of 0.4 mm of the labial bone thickness was observed between implant placement and the second-stage surgery.

CAN WE PREDICT BONE RESORPTION OR THE LACK THEREOF?

There is no evidence on how to predict bone resorption of the labial bone after tooth removal. When there is less than 1.0 mm thickness of labial bone then the clinician should expect some of its loss. In such situations, grafting a relatively nonresorbable material may be indicated. If there is extremely thick bone, for example, greater than 1.5 mm thickness, the clinician may believe that this bone will not resorb; however, there is minimal evidence in the literature to support this claim. The author always expects bone to resorb to some degree, and tries to perform adjunctive procedures to anticipate its resorption and a resultant flatter ridge form.

Do Existing Bone Defects on the Labial Surface Affect Gingival Position?

Kan and colleagues[12] looked at this question in a small sample of patients, and concluded that as the size and shape of the labial bone defect increased, there was a greater incidence of gingival recession above 1.5 mm. 8.3% of V-shaped defects, 42.8% of U-shaped defects, and 100% of large-shaped defects had greater than 1.5 mm of gingival recession.

When a tooth is removed and a facial defect exists, the clinician may graft the defect. However, the material chosen must perform several tasks, the first of which is to promote bone formation within the extraction defect to later support an implant. The second is to achieve minimal resorption to promote preservation or recreation of the normal convex ridge profile. Allograft is often chosen because of its reported success with bone formation within 4 months of placement. However, at 4 months and over time, further bone remodeling will often occur with a resultant flattened ridge. In the critical esthetic defect, additional onlay application of a relatively nonresorbable material such as anorganic bovine bone may be necessary to recreate the desired ridge form. Another solution when smaller ridge form corrections are needed is the conversion of thin gingiva to thick gingiva with the placement of a connective tissue graft.

What is the Effect of Gingival Thickness on Maintenance of the Facial Gingival Margin Over Time?

It was noticed as early as 1969, and confirmed, that patients with thin gingiva have gingival recession after osseous surgery around teeth. Patients with thicker gingiva had pocket formation without gingival recession after osseous surgery, simultaneous with crestal bone resorption.[14–16]

Kan and colleagues[10] reported a series of patients who had subepithelial connective tissue grafts placed under their gingiva on the labial surface of implant sites to change the patients' thin gingiva to thick gingiva. This conversion resulted in less gingival recession over time. Although this was a relatively small series of patients, this observation has been confirmed by the author. Kan states: "facial gingival recession of thin periodontal biotype seems to be more pronounced than that of thick biotype. Biotype conversion around both natural teeth and implants with subepithelial connective tissue graft has been advocated, and the resulting tissues appear to be more resistant to recession."[10] Based on these observations, if a tooth in the esthetic region has thin gingiva at the crest, a connective tissue graft should be placed under the gingiva to convert it form thin to thick, resulting in thickened tissue with a better appearance. It also provides the restorative dentist with sufficient tissue to mold and sculpt with prosthetic manipulation.

Implant design may contribute to the ability of clinicians to maintain the position of the facial gingival margin. It is well accepted that a flat, butt joint between the abutment and implant will result in a 1.0-mm dimension inflammatory zone. This zone will adversely affect bone and its movement away from the inflamed area of tissue, resulting in 2 to 3 mm of bone loss from the implant/abutment interface. To circumvent this phenomenon, manufacturers have medialized the interface utilizing internal connections of the abutment to implant, resulting in an average of 0.5 mm crestal bone loss. Of importance, this lack of bone movement in the apical direction results in preservation of the bone around the implant. Bone preservation is circumferential with maintenance of the facial crestal bone, with subsequent less gingival recession because the crestal bone is maintained over time.[17–19]

Papilla are directly influenced by the underlying bone. If the bone on the adjacent tooth is within 5 to 6 mm of the contact area of the teeth, papilla will usually be normal in appearance. If the crestal bone on the adjacent tooth has undergone resorption then the papilla may be blunted with significant defects noted. The facial gingival margin is not directly influenced by the interdental bone unless the bone loss around the tooth before its removal and the bone levels on the adjacent teeth have been compromised prior to tooth removal.[20–22]

The facial gingival margin level will also be influenced by the methods used immediately after tooth removal. In an clinical trial supported by the National Institutes of Health,[23] it was found that placing an abutment immediately on the implant at time of implant placement at the same time as tooth removal resulted in more facial gingival tissue preservation as compared with a delayed procedure. Patients in the delayed group had the tooth removed and the socket grafted. After 4 months elapsed, the implant was placed with a provisional restoration. In this group the facial gingival margin was 1 mm more apical compared with the immediate provisionalized group. The immediate provisionalized group had the tooth removed with immediate implant and provisional crown placement. The immediate provisionalized group had 1 mm more coronal tissue than the delayed group.

Based on the foregoing discussion, an algorithm for treatment can be formed (**Figs. 1–4**).

The clinician should assess the bone and soft tissue of the patient, and establish the ideal location of the facial gingival margin.

At the time of tooth removal:

1. If there is a lack of labial bone, the site should be grafted with a material that will form bone within the socket for later implant placement. The clinician should consider the need for a subepithelial connective tissue graft to convert thin to thick gingiva. After the graft heals, one must consider placing the implant with simultaneous insertion of a healing abutment or provisional restoration to maintain the position of the facial gingival margin.
2. If there is intact labial bone or very minimal labial bone defects, the clinician should place the implant immediately after tooth removal, if there is no purulent exudate. The tooth is removed with complete preservation of the labial bone, the implant is

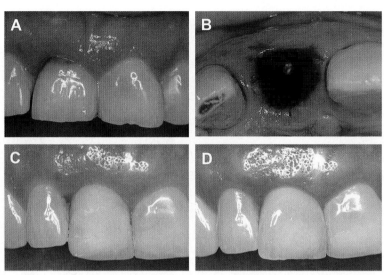

Fig. 1. (*A*) Preextraction view of right central incisor. Note the presence of thick gingiva and that the facial gingival margin is at an ideal position. (*B*) The tooth is removed and the implant sit prepared. The labial bone was intact. The implant is positioned palatal to the incisor edge. No additional grafting is necessary. (*C*) A provisional restoration was placed immediately after implant position. Note the preservation of the vertical position of the facial gingival margin. (*D*) The final restoration 2 years after initial restoration shows maintenance of the position of the facial gingival margin.

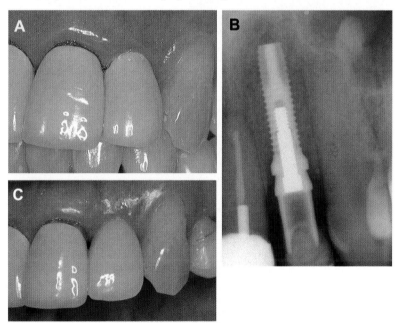

Fig. 2. (*A*) Preextraction view of the left lateral incisor. The facial gingival margin position is ideal. The labial bone thickness is marginal and the tissue is not thick. (*B*) After the tooth was removed an implant was placed with a provisional. The implant utilized a medialized abutment implant interface to preserve the presence of the facial bone. This 4-month post-restoration radiograph shows excellent bone preservation. (*C*) The final restoration shows excellent maintenance of the position of the facial gingival margin.

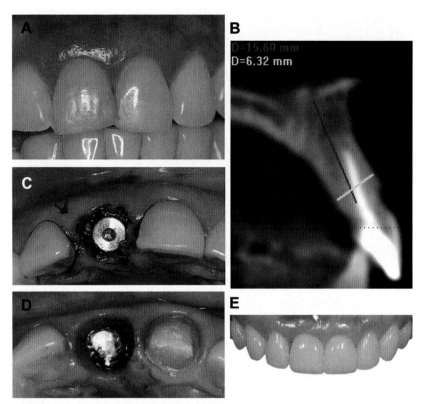

Fig. 3. (A) This patient has a fractured right central incisor. The tooth length is 10.5 mm and the gingiva is medium thickness. The facial gingival margin is in an ideal position. (B) The cross section shows thin labial bone. (C) The tooth was removed with preservation of the thin labial bone. The implant was placed and the gap between the implant surface, and the intact labial bone was grafted with bovine particulate graft material. A healing abutment was placed to aid in preservation of the level of the facial gingival margin. (D) This view shows the preservation of the gingival thickness with mild flattening of the horizontal projection of the crest. The final restoration will aid in moving the gingival projection to ideal morphology. (E) The final restoration with preservation of the original position of the facial gingival margin.

placed, the space between the implant and intact labial bone is grafted with a bovine particulate xenograft, and a healing abutment is placed. If necessary a connective tissue graft can be placed after the implant site has healed to further augment the horizontal appearance of the gingival complex. This method preserves ridge contour and preserves the level of the facial gingival margin.

3. If the facial gingival margin on the tooth prior to removal is apical to the ideal location, diagnosed from a presurgical mockup, then treatment should be considered to move the gingival margin coronally. The clinician should consider orthodontic extrusion.[24] The tooth is orthodontically extruded to move the gingival margin coronally. The tooth is removed following the protocol suggested by Brindis and Block.[24]

4. When possible, the clinician should place a healing abutment to maintain the facial gingival margin height. If the gingival margin is held in its original position, it will

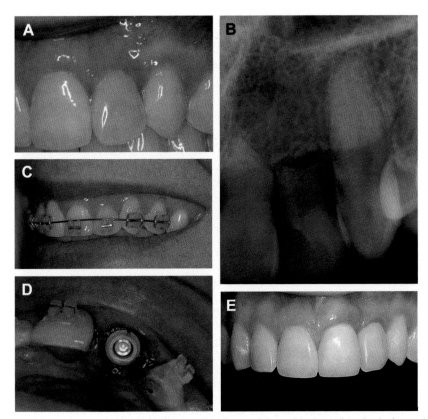

Fig. 4. (*A*) Preextraction view of left central incisor and lateral incisor. The gingival margins are 1 mm apical to ideal and the gingiva is thin. (*B*) This radiograph shows severe resorption of the roots of the left central incisor and lateral incisor. (*C*) Orthodontic extrusion was performed to move the facial gingival margin coronally before tooth removal. The gingival margin was overcorrected 2 mm coronal to the final desired position. (*D*) The teeth were removed in 2 visits to preserve interdental bone. The tooth was removed, the implant was placed, bovine graft material was placed between the implant and the labial bone, and a zirconium healing abutment placed. These procedures were performed to idealize the form of the crest and maintain the position of the gingival margin. (*E*) The final crowns show maintenance of the facial gingival margin and crestal ridge width.

recede less than if allowed to flatten when the implant is not placed or of a cover screw is placed subgingivally.[23]

5. In the esthetic implant site, more apical movement of the facial gingival margin will occur if the bone and soft tissue is thin or lacking.

REFERENCES

1. Panossian AJ, Block MS. Evaluation of the smile: facial and dental considerations. J Oral Maxillofac Surg 2010;68(3):547–54.
2. Sarver D, Jacobson RS. The aesthetic dentofacial analysis. Clin Plast Surg 2007; 34(3):369–94.
3. Sarver DM. The importance of incisor positioning in the esthetic smile: the smile arc. Am J Orthod Dentofacial Orthop 2001;120:98–111.

4. Vig RG, Brundo GC. The kinetics of anterior tooth display. J Prosthet Dent 1978; 39:502–4.
5. Ash MM, Nelson S, editors. Wheeler's dental anatomy chart, in wheeler's dental anatomy, physiology, and occlusion. 8th edition. Philadelphia: W.B. Saunders; 2003. p. 35.
6. Goldstein RE, Goldstein CE. Is your case really finished? In: Bell WH, editor. Modern practice in orthognathic and reconstructive surgery. Philadelphia: W.B. Saunders Company; 1992. p. 219–33. Chapter 8 (43).
7. Allen EP, Bell WH, Garber DH. Achieving the esthetic smile. In: Bell WH, editor. Modern practice in orthognathic and reconstructive surgery. Philadelphia: W.B. Saunders Company; 1992. p. 235–61. Chapter 9.
8. Kan JY, Morimoto T, Rungcharassaeng K, et al. Gingival biotype assessment in the esthetic zone: visual versus direct measurement. Int J Periodontics Restorative Dent 2010;30(3):237–43.
9. Kan JY, Rungcharassaeng K, Morimoto T, et al. Facial gingival tissue stability after connective tissue graft with single immediate tooth replacement in the esthetic zone: consecutive case report. J Oral Maxillofac Surg 2009;67(Suppl 11): 40–8.
10. Kan JY, Rungcharassaeng K, Lozada JL. Bilaminar subepithelial connective tissue grafts for immediate implant placement and provisionalization in the esthetic zone. J Calif Dent Assoc 2005;33(11):865–71.
11. Cardaropoli G, Lekholm U, Wennstrom JL. Tissue alterations at implant-supported single-tooth replacements: a 1-year prospective clinical study. Clin Oral Implants Res 2006;17(2):165–71.
12. Kan JY, Rungcharassaeng K, Sclar A, et al. Effects of the facial osseous defect morphology on gingival dynamics after immediate tooth replacement and guided bone regeneration: 1-year results. J Oral Maxillofac Surg 2007;65(7 Suppl 1): 13–9 Erratum appears in J Oral Maxillofac Surg 2008;66(10):2195–6.
13. Block MS, Kent JN. A comparison of particulate and solid root forms of hydroxylapatite in dog extraction sites. J Oral Maxillofac Surg 1986;44:89–93.
14. Ochsenbein C, Ross S. A reevaluation of osseous surgery. Dent Clin North Am 1969;13(1):87–102.
15. Weisgold AS. Contours of the full crown restoration. Alpha Omegan 1977;70(3): 77–89.
16. Ochsenbein C, Ross S. A concept of osseous surgery and its clinical application. In: Ward HL, editor. A periodontal point of view. Philadephia: WB Saunders, Charles C. Thomas; 1973. Chapter 13.
17. Atieh MA, Ibrahim HM, Atieh AH. Platform switching for marginal bone preservation around dental implants: a systemic review and meta-analysis. J Periodontol 2010;81(10):1350–66.
18. Wagenberg B, Froum SJ. Prospective study of 94 platform-switched implants observed from 1992 to 2006. Int J Periodontics Restorative Dent 2010;30(1):9–17.
19. Baumgarten H. Preservation of crestal bone: a clinical requisite. Pract Proced Aesthet Dent 2006;18(7):431–2.
20. Ryser MR, Block MS, Mercante DE. Correlation of papilla to crestal bone levels around single tooth implants in immediate or delayed crown protocols. J Oral Maxillofac Surg 2005;63(8):1184–95.
21. Tarnow DP, Magner AW, Fletcher P. The effect of the distance from the contact point to the crest of bone on the presence or absence of the interproximal dental papilla. J Periodontol 1992;63(12):995–6.

22. Tarnow D, Elian N, Fletcher P, et al. Vertical distance from the crest of bone to the height of the interproximal papilla between adjacent implants. J Periodontol 2003; 74(12):1785–8.
23. Block MS, Mercante DE, Lirette D, et al. Prospective evaluation of immediate and delayed provisional single tooth restorations. J Oral Maxillofac Surg 2009; 67(Suppl 11):89–107.
24. Brindis MA, Block MS. Orthodontic toot extrusion to enhance soft tissue implant esthetics. J Oral Maxillofac Surg 2009;67(Suppl 11):49–59.

Bone Grafting the Mandible

Patrick J. Louis, DDS, MD

KEYWORDS

• Bone grafting • Mandible • Dentate • Edentulous

Multiple bone grafting techniques have been used to reconstruct the partially dentate and edentulous mandible.[1–6] Many of these techniques have been successful. In this article, the various bone grafting techniques to reconstruct mandibular defects are reviewed. Other issues discussed include whether autogenous bone is necessary for reconstruction of the mandibular ridge and the importance of membranes.

BLOCK ONLAY GRAFTS

Block onlay grafts have been used extensively for reconstruction of mandibular alveolar defects.[7–11] Autogenous and nonautogenous options are available for vertical and horizontal deficiencies of the mandible. Autogenous bone grafts have the advantage of transferring osteogenic cells to the recipient site.[12–15] Autogenous donor sites for block grafts include the calvarium, mandible, zygoma, and ilium. Intramembranous bone (calvarium, mandible, and zygoma) has the advantage of decreased rates of resorption compared with endochondral bone (ilium), due to its dense cortical structure and microarchitecture.[16–20]

When a small amount of bone is needed, local grafts harvested from the mandibular symphysis or ramus have been used extensively (**Fig. 1**).[10,21–24] These sources have the advantage of being convenient due to their proximity to the reconstruction site and low risk of morbidity.[25] The disadvantage of the mandible as a bone source is the limited amount of bone available and the fact that mandibular harvesting can sometimes interfere with the planned reconstruction if too close to the reconstruction site (**Table 1**).[26] The most common postoperative morbidity associated with chin and ramus grafts has been reported as temporary paresthesia. For the chin it ranges from 10% to 50%, and for the ramus, it ranges from 0% to 5%.[21,27] The zygomaticomaxillary region also can be used as a harvest site.[28] The advantage of this site is that when performing grafts in the maxilla, simple extension of the incision is needed. The procedure is associated with a low risk of morbidity. The disadvantage is the

This article was previously published in the May 2011 issue of *Oral and Maxillofacial Surgery Clinics of North America*.
Oral and Maxillofacial Surgery, School of Dentistry, University of Alabama at Birmingham, 1919 7th Avenue South, SDB 419, Birmingham, AL 35294, USA
E-mail address: plouis@uab.edu

Dent Clin N Am 55 (2011) 673–695
doi:10.1016/j.cden.2011.07.006
dental.theclinics.com

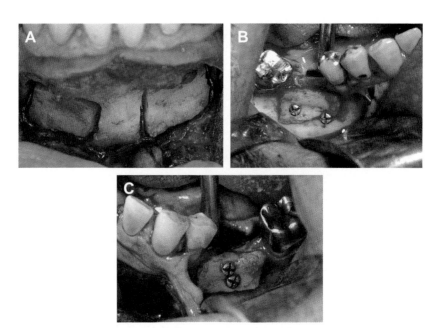

Fig. 1. (A) Harvest of block graft from the symphysis of the mandible. (B) Horizontal augmentation of the posterior mandible with block graft. (C) Horizontal augmentation of the posterior mandible with block graft.

limited amount of bone available. Other sites that can be used are the maxillary tuberosity and tori.[29–31]

Distant site bone harvesting is indicated when a large graft is needed (see **Table 1**).[5,8,17,32–36] Sites that have been reported as reliable include the calvarium and the ilium (**Fig. 2**). The tibia can be used for harvesting cancellous bone; however, a small amount of block cortical bone also can be harvested.[37,38] When cancellous bone is needed, the tibia is chosen, because it yields an abundant amount with a relatively low risk of morbidity.[39–41]

Table 1
Donor sites for bone grafting with published bone volumes

Donor Site	Noncompressed Corticocancellous (mL)	Block (cm)	References
Symphysis	4.71	2.09 × 0.99 × 0.69	Montazem et al,[113] 2000
Ascending Ramus	2.36	3.76 × 3.32 × 2.25 × 0.92	Gungormus et al,[114,115] 2002
Lateral Ramus	NA (not available)	1.3 × 3	Li and Schwartz,[116] 1996
Cornoid Process	NA	1.8 × 1.7 × 0.5	Choung and Kim,[117] 2001
Zygomatic Butress	NA	1.5 × 2	Gellrich et al,[28] 2007
Tiba	20–40	1 × 2	Caytone et al,[39] 1992
Anterior Ilium	50	1 × 3	Marx and Morales,[49] 1988
Posterior Ilium	100–125	5 × 5	Marx and Morales,[49] 1988
Calvarium	NA	NA	Moreira-Gonzalez et al,[43] 2006

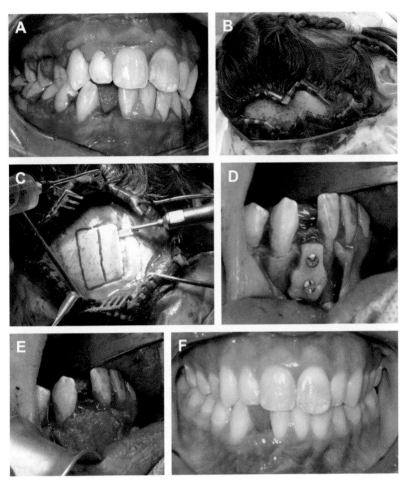

Fig. 2. (*A*) Clinical photograph of a patient who had avulsion of one of the mandibular incisors secondary to a motor vehicle accident. (*B*) Scalp incision for access to the calvarium. (*C*) Outline and harvest of block graft from the outer table of the right parietal bone for reconstruction. (*D*) Block graft for augmentation of the anterior mandible. (*E*) Particulate autogenous bone graft has been placed over the block graft and will be covered with a membrane. (*F*) Postoperative view of bone graft site with excellent bone contour. Note the fixation screw is visible through the mucosa. (*G*) Implant placement after exposure of the augmented site. (*H*) Restored mandibular incisor immediately after final restoration. Note the excellent ridge contour. (*I*) Restored mandibular incisor several months after final restoration placed.

The types of grafts harvested from the calvarium and the ilium are entirely different. Calvarial grafts are usually harvested in strips from the parietal bone. The average thickness of the parietal bone is 7.45 mm.[42,43] A split thickness harvest technique is used, which can yield graft thicknesses of approximately 3 mm. The main advantage of calvarial grafts is their dense cortical structure that resists resorption.[16–18] The amount of available cortical graft is abundant. However, this procedure usually requires general anesthesia in a hospital or ambulatory care setting, but there are a few reports of office based techniques.[44,45] The incidence of complication is low,

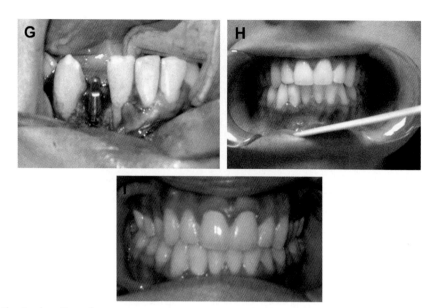

Fig. 2. (*continued*)

with the most common reported complication being seroma/hematoma.[46] Larger amounts of bone can be harvested from the ilium, but these grafts typically have a thin cortical layer and a thick cancellous portion.[35,47] The main advantages of these grafts are the large volume of bone that can be harvested and carved into various shapes.[48,49] The main disadvantage is the morbidity associated with bone graft harvest. The reported complication incidence is higher than with other donor sites. Reported complications include gait disturbance, paresthesia, hematoma/seroma, and fracture.[49–53]

Horizontal Segmental Defects

These cases have adequate alveolar bone height but inadequate width. The deficiency is most commonly on the facial surface of the mandible. The planning of these cases should include physical and radiographic examination. The site and the planned implant diameter dictate the amount of bone required. In the mandibular incisor, region a 3 mm diameter implant is usually indicated. The amount of bone needed is 1 mm to 1.5 mm of bone on both the facial and lingual aspect of the implant. Thus, in the incisor region, the minimum amount of bone needed is 4 mm to 5 mm. In the canine and premolar region, the usual implant diameter is approximately 4 mm, and the width of bone needed is 6 mm to 7 mm. In the molar region, the approximate size of the implant needed is usually 5 mm, and the minimum width required is 7 mm to 8 mm. When grafting these various sites, the thickness of the block graft should be slightly larger than the final planned width.

For most segmental deficiencies in the mandible, autogenous grafts can be harvested from the symphysis or ramus. The planned recipient site is usually exposed through a crestal incision. Depending on location of the deficiency, the donor site may be accessed through extension of this incision. Once the site is exposed, the defect can be measured and the size of the bone graft determined.

Many surgeons choose to use a piezoelectric drill because of its versatility.[54–58] Both the donor site and the recipient site require preparation. The graft, once harvested, is tried into position to determine where trimming is needed. The facial surface of the recipient site is usually flattened, as is the surface of the graft that will be in contact with the recipient site. This allows for more intimate contact between the two surfaces and better incorporation of the graft. Once the desired shape is achieved, the graft is set into position, and depending on the size of the graft, secured into position with 1–2 resorbable or titanium screws.[59,60] Gaps between the bone graft and the recipient site are filled with particulate bone and covered with a resorbable or nonresorbable membrane. Primary closure is achieved, and the graft is allowed to heal for 3 to 4 months before implant placement.

With larger segments of deficient bone, multiple local sites can be harvested or a distant site can be chosen. The calvarium or ilium can be used but should be chosen based on the application needed. In the case of horizontal deficiency, that is 3 mm or less, the calvarium would be a good choice. When more horizontal augmentation is needed, the ilium could be used or particulate graft added along the buccal or facial aspect of the graft. The block graft is secured with screws, and the entire graft is covered with a membrane. Primary closure is achieved with 4(0) Vicryl (Ethicon Incorporated, Somerville, NJ, USA) or Monocryl (Ethicon Incorporated, Somerville, NJ, USA).

Horizontal Deficiency of the Mandibular Arch

The edentulous horizontally deficient mandible can be treated with multiple local grafts or bone from distant sites. Because of the large amount of bone needed, harvest from a distant site is usually indicated. Exposure is usually performed through a vestibular incision. The mental nerves are identified and protected. Once the alveolus is encountered, the incision is carried through the periosteum, and the ridge is exposed. The grafts are mortised into position by preparing both the recipient site and bone graft. Once a good fit is ensured, the graft is secured into position with screws. The graft is protected with a membrane, and the wound is closed primarily.

Vertical Segmental Defects

Vertical augmentation of the alveolar ridge is more difficult than horizontal augmentation. There is concern when expanding the soft tissue envelope vertically there is an increased risk of graft exposure. A second concern is the adequate adaptation of the bone graft, which is critical for graft success.

Many of these alveolar ridges are deficient in height and width and may require flattening for better graft adaptation. If thin cortical grafts are harvested, then a stack technique is used to achieve the desired result. This technique involves the mortising of the graft to the ridge surface and the placement of multiple block grafts stacked on one another to achieve height. The graft is secured with a bone screw or by dental implants. A second technique is to augment the defect with a single corticocancellous block that adequately replaces the desired amount of bone.

Segmental defects are usually exposed through a crestal incision. Once good bone adaptation is achieved between the graft and recipient site, the graft is secured with titanium screws. Any gaps between the recipient site and the bone graft are filled with particulate bone graft and covered with a membrane. To achieve closure of the wound, the periosteum of the flap is released. This is achieved by placing a horizontal incision just through the periosteum under the flap. This allows the flap to stretch and permits primary closure without wound tension.

Vertical Deficiency of the Mandibular Arch

This generally requires a large amount of autogenous bone from the calvarium or the ilium. As discussed earlier, reconstruction can be performed using a stacked calvarial graft that is shaped and mortised to the desired height (**Fig. 3**). Iliac crest grafts do not require stacking; instead the ridge is exposed through a vestibular incision, the mental nerves identified, the block secured with titanium screws, and gaps filled with cancellous particulate, then covered with a membrane before performing a 2-layer closure.

Allogeneic Block Grafts

Allogeneic block grafts have not had extensive use in implant dentistry.[61–63] A systemic review of the literature by Waasdorp identified 35 papers, with only nine publications meeting inclusion criteria (2 case reports, 6 case series, and 1 prospective, multicenter, consecutive case series).[64] There were no randomized controlled clinical trials identified. Observational studies generally report graft incorporation rates of 90% or greater and implant survival of 99% to 100%. The shortcomings of these studies is that most reports involved selected defects in anterior regions and had short term follow-ups of less than 3 years. The reviewers concluded that case-based reports document the potential for allogeneic block grafts to support alveolar ridge

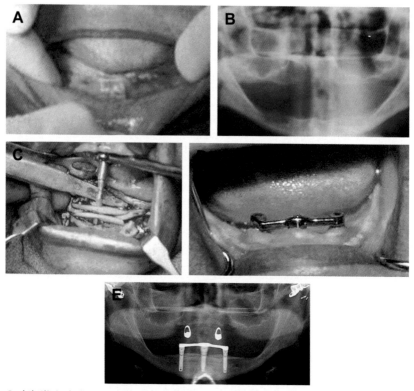

Fig. 3. (A) Clinical photograph of atrophic mandible. (B) Preoperative panoramic radiograph. (C) Vertical augmentation of the mandibular ridge with calvarial bone and simultaneous implant placement. (D) Long-term follow-up of the restored ridge. (E) 10-year follow-up radiograph showing excellent incorporation of the bone graft and excellent long-term stability.

augmentation and implant placement, but there is insufficient evidence to establish treatment efficacy relative to graft incorporation, alveolar ridge augmentation, and long-term dental implant survival.

Allogeneic block grafts can be substituted for autogenous grafts to avoid donor site morbidity, but the risk of exposure is higher, especially with vertical augmentation.[61]

BARRIER MEMBRANES

Barrier membranes have been studied extensively in the dental and maxillofacial literature.[27,65–73] Membranes have been shown to protect both block and particulate onlay grafts.[74] The surgeon has the choice of resorbable versus nonresorbable and rigid versus nonrigid membranes when performing grafting procedures. Studies suggest that there is less resorption of block and particulate grafts when a membrane remains in place throughout the healing phase of the graft.[74,75] Significant resorption can occur for block grafts left unprotected, but not always.[76] Vertical augmentation is particularly problematic with both block and particulate grafts, with resorption rates that have been reported higher than for horizontal augmentation.[76] Cordaro reported resorption rates of 23.5% for lateral augmentation and 42% for vertical augmentation when using block grafts without a membrane.[76] Particulate onlay grafts can undergo even more resorption.[75]

Block grafts have structural integrity and thus maintain space and resist resorption.[17,18] Particulate grafts lack structural integrity and can be displaced.[75] With horizontal augmentation, where the vertical height is adequate and only width is lacking, particulate graft material can be used and protected with a membrane. The choice of particulate graft material becomes important if a nonrigid membrane is used. The particulate graft must have some strength to resist deformation by the soft tissue envelope.[75,77] In this case, it is preferable to use a mineralized bone product such as autogenous bone, mineralized allogeneic bone, or anorganic bovine bone. If a rigid membrane is used, then the choice of material becomes less crucial, as a rigid membrane will maintain space and protect the graft.[78–80]

When vertical augmentation is indicated, block or particulate graft can be chosen. If a block graft is chosen, it has the advantage of structural integrity to maintain space; however, because of high resorption potential, membrane protection is warranted.[74,76] A nonrigid, resorbable or nonresorbable membrane can be used.

When a particulate graft is selected for vertical augmentation, a rigid membrane must be used to protect the graft. The technique of vertical augmentation with particulate grafts protected by a rigid membrane has been reported to be successful.[78,79,81] These techniques have been associated with a high rate of exposure that can negatively affect the graft. Exposure rates are as high as 50%, particularly when large vertical augmentations are performed.[78] One of the techniques that has been described to minimize graft exposure is the use of PRP (platelet-rich plasma gel) placed over the rigid membrane before wound closure.[82]

PARTICULATE GRAFTS

Particulate onlay grafts have been used extensively for reconstruction of mandibular alveolar defects. Autogenous and nonautogenous options are available. The source of autogenous particulate is the same as has been discussed for block harvest (see **Table 1**). For small amounts of bone, local sites can be used, including the symphysis, ramus, and maxillary tuberosity. This is usually harvested with a bone shaver. When greater volumes of bone are needed, then distant sites are employed. Particulate grafts have the advantage of rapid vascularization, but they must be protected by a membrane to reduce the risk of resorption.

Allogeneic and xenogenic particulate grafts have been growing in popularity. These grafts are readily available and abundant. They can be used in combination with autogenous bone or alone. Recent studies have shown success with these graft materials for vertical ridge augmentation when protected with a rigid membrane.[82,83]

Segmental Horizontal Defects

The reconstruction of the partially edentulous mandible with particulate graft material can be performed with various bone graft materials. The type of graft material needed will depend on the size of the defect and type of membrane used. With horizontal augmentation, where the vertical height is adequate, and only width is lacking, particulate graft material can be used and protected with a membrane (**Fig. 4**). When a mineralized bone graft is used, a nonrigid membrane is suggested. In this technique, the graft is placed through a crestal incision. The defect is grafted, then protected with membrane. If a rigid membrane is used, it must be fixed with screws. If a nonrigid membrane is used, the edges of the membrane must be tucked and secured underneath the flap.

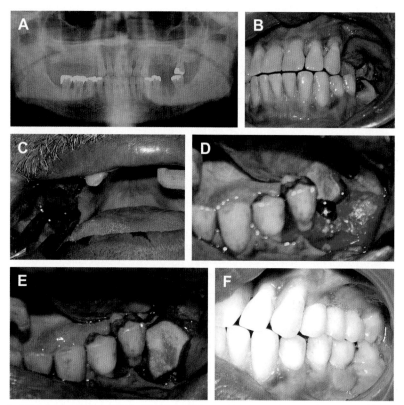

Fig. 4. (*A*) Preoperative radiograph of a patient missing tooth #30. This site has adequate height but not width. (*B*) Preoperative photograph. (*C*) Harvest of bone during a right maxillary tuberosity reduction. (*D, E*) Horizontal augmentation of the right posterior mandible during implant placement. (*F*) Final restoration in place, area #30.

Demineralized bone graft materials tend to be soft and easily compressed by the soft tissue envelope. If only demineralized product is used to augment a horizontal defect, a rigid membrane should be used to protect the graft. This membrane must be secured with screws to the underlying bone to prevent micromotion. To close the wound, a periosteal releasing incision may be required. The particulate graft must have some strength to resist deformation. In this case, it is preferable to use mineralized product such as autogenous bone, mineralized allogeneic bone, or anorganic bovine bone as the graft of choice. However, if a rigid membrane is used, then the choice of material becomes less crucial.

The technique is done through a vestibular incision to expose the edentulous space. The incision is extended to near the junction of the attached mucosa. Mobilization of the facial, crestal, and lingual aspect of the soft tissues is usually performed. The dissection around the cervical portion of the teeth is performed in a tunneling fashion subperiosteally to mobilize the gingival cuff. As an alternative to a vestibular incision, a crestal incision can be used in conjunction with releasing incision at least 2 teeth on either side of the defect. Once the ridge is exposed, a titanium mesh membrane can be trimmed and contoured to fit into position as a crib. This is then filled with bone graft and secured with at least 2 screws on the facial aspect. When a crestal incision is used for exposure, the periosteum must be released along the facial vestibule to facilitate a tension-free closure of the wound. This is usually not necessary when a vestibular incision is used. Closure is performed in layers with 3.0 Vicyrl suture material placed deep to the mucosa. The mucosa is closed with 4.0 Vicyrl or Monocryl suture.

Segmental Vertical Defects

When using a particulate bone graft for vertical ridge augmentation, a rigid membrane must be used to prevent deformation and resorption of the graft. The reconstruction is performed in similar fashion as described in the section Segmental Horizontal Defects (Fig. 5).

Horizontal Deficiency of the Mandibular Arch

To reconstruct horizontal deficiency of the mandibular alveolus with particulate graft, the principles of graft protection during the healing phase are important. The ridge is exposed through a vestibular incision. After identification of the mental nerves, the dissection is carried toward the ridge. The periosteum is incised, and a subperiosteal dissection is performed to expose the ridge. The particulate graft is placed and then covered with a membrane. The choice of particulate graft material becomes important if a nonrigid membrane is used. The particulate graft must have some strength to resist deformation.[75,77] In this case, it is preferable to use mineralized bone as the graft of choice. If a rigid membrane is used, the choice of material becomes less crucial, as a rigid membrane will maintain space and protect the graft. Following membrane placement, the wound is closed primarily.[78–80]

Vertical Deficiency of the Mandibular Arch

When augmenting the highly atrophic edentulous mandible vertically, an intraoral or extraoral approach can be used. The intraoral approach is more straightforward. In this technique, an incision is made in the depth of the mandibular vestibule just anterior to the retromolar pad extending anteriorly across the midline. After identifying and protecting the mental nerves, a subperiosteal dissection is achieved. In the extremely atrophic mandible, the inferior alveolar nerve may be exposed along the crest due to dehiscence of the canal. In this case, a preferred technique is to start anteriorly and identify the mental foramina and then dissect posteriorly. With this technique, the

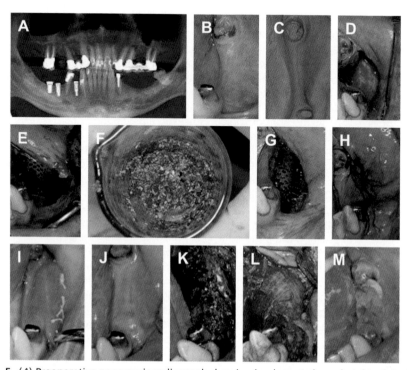

Fig. 5. (*A*) Preoperative panoramic radiograph showing inadequate bone height of the left posterior mandible. (*B*) Preoperative view of the narrow posterior mandibular ridge. (*C*) Preoperative cast. (*D*) Exposure of the posterior mandible through a vestibular incision. (*E*) Try in of the titanium mesh. (*F*) Mineralized and demineralized bone mixture. (*G*) Augmentation of the posterior mandibular ridge with allogeneic bone and titanium mesh. (*H*) Soft tissue flap draped over the mesh. (*I*) Posterior alveolar ridge 1 week postoperatively. (*J*) Posterior alveolar ridge 4 months postoperatively. (*K*) Surgical exposure of the ridge. (*L*) After removal of the mesh there is excellent bone height and width. (*M*) Surgical guide in place. (*N*) Panoramic radiograph 4 months postoperatively. (*O*) Cone-beam computed tomography (CT) scan showing a cross-sectional view of the posterior ridge at 4 months. Note the excellent bone height and width. (*P*) Mirror view of the alveolar ridge with implants in place. (*Q*) Postoperative radiograph with implants in place. (*R*) Final restoration in place.

dissection is carried onto the lingual surface of the mandible in a subperiosteal fashion. The lingual extent of the dissection anteriorly is to the genial tubercles. The genioglossus and geniohyoid should not be detached.

Once the mandible is exposed, the preferred technique for vertical augmentation is the use of preformed titanium mesh. A right hemi-tray and left hemi-tray are chosen based on the desired level of augmentation. This is determined by preoperative planning with study models and radiographs. The mesh is contoured and trimmed to fit. Relief over the mental foramina is necessary to avoid injury to the nerve. It is desirable to extend the mesh to the posterior aspect of the mandible in the region of the retromolar pad, as the crest of the ridge begins to turn superiorly to form the ramus. This is done to avoid any sharp areas at the end of the mesh that may later become exposed. In patients with larger mandibles, two trays may not be long enough to extend posteriorly to the retromolar region while still covering the anterior aspect of the mandible. In

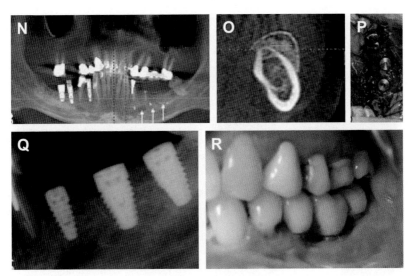

Fig. 5. (*continued*)

these cases, a third piece of titanium mesh must be contoured and overlapped onto the anterior aspects of both hemi-trays in order to protect the graft that will be placed in this location.

The mesh is filled with the bone graft and secured into position with at least 2 screws on the facial surface of each hemi-tray and 1 screw on the lingual, usually in the anterior region just above the genial tubercles. If an additional midline mesh is needed to cover the graft, it can be secured on the facial and lingual of the ridge. PRP gel can be placed over the mesh before closure of the incision to minimize exposure. Because the incision is made in the vestibule, the soft tissue is thick and should be closed in two layers.

An extraoral approach also can be used when augmenting the mandible (**Figs. 6 and 7**). This approach is more difficult than an intraoral approach because it involves transposition of the inferior alveolar nerves. This incision is made under sterile conditions along the submental crease. The incision must be extended along the full length of the submental crease in order to achieve adequate exposure. This dissection is carried sharply down to the inferior border of the mandible where a subperiosteal dissection is performed to expose the facial and superior aspect of the mandible. From this approach, the mental nerves can be easily identified. When there is a dehiscence of the inferior alveolar nerve, the neurovascular bundle is mobilized and transposed posteriorly. In cases where there is no dehiscence, the inferior alveolar nerve transposition is performed in order to achieve adequate mobilization of the mental nerve and provide room for the bone graft and titanium mesh trays. Once the inferior alveolar nerve is transposed, usually to the second molar region, the titanium mesh tray can be contoured and trimmed.

The posterior extent of the inferior aspect of the tray should be placed just anterior to the exit of the inferior alveolar neurovascular bundle. The superior aspect of the tray can extend posteriorly to the retromolar region. The mucosa must be fully mobilized in the retromolar pad region and on the lingual aspect of the mandible to prevent pinching or tearing of the mucosa when the titanium mesh is inserted. Once the mesh has been properly contoured and fitted, it is filled with the particulate bone graft and secured as described previously. PRP is placed and the wound closed.

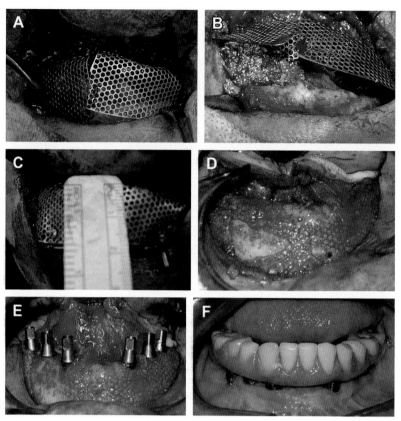

Fig. 6. (*A*) Submental approach to the atrophic mandible. Pre-formed titanium trays have being tried in and trimmed. (*B*) The particulate bone graft is being placed into the site. (*C*) Measurement of the trays that are in place shows a height of around 20 mm. (*D*) Postoperative view of the augmented mandible after 6 months of healing. (*E*) Implant placement. (*F*) Final restoration at 2-year follow-up.

During wound closure, the soft tissue is redraped into position, the vestibule deepened using a suturing technique described by Bosker using 2.0 Vicryl suture placed in a submucosal fashion at the desired depth of the vestibule.[83] This is sutured inferiorly to the periosteum and musculature along the inferior lingual aspect of the mandible. The second layer is placed at the level of the mentalis muscle superiorly and secured to the digastric musculature. The platysma muscle is then closed. In most patients, some of the overlying skin along the incision can be excised in a lazy W fashion in order to improve neck contour.[84,85] This suturing technique will roll the lower lip outward and give the lip a more full appearance.

INLAY BONE GRAFTS

The osteomucoperiosteal flap can be used along with inlay bone grafting to reconstruct mandibular segmental alveolar defects or entire arch deficiencies. The osteoperiosteal flap, for the purposes of this discussion, is defined as a vascularized segmental osteotomy of alveolar bone, applied in order to expand the alveolus vertically or horizontally. The procedure has the distinct advantage of being a vascularized

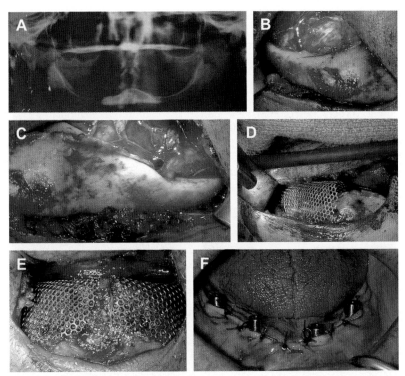

Fig. 7. (*A*) Preoperative panoramic radiograph of a patient with severe mandibular atrophy. (*B*) View of the right posterior mandible. (*C*) View of the left posterior mandible. Note the severe atrophy. (*D*) Titanium mesh try in. (*E*) Particulate bone graft in place, contained with titanium mesh. (*F*) Implants in the reconstructed ridge at 10 months after ridge reconstruction.

flap in which the bone that is being transported maintains its own blood supply from attached soft tissue. Vascularized bone transport has a rich history in oral and maxillofacial surgery and is performed routinely in orthognathic surgery.[86–91] The research on the blood supply of osteotomized segments when performing orthognathic surgery has been well studied.[92–96] Studies on small segment osteotomies have shown similar results as studies on Le Fort I osteotomies. Revascularization usually occurs within 2 weeks.[95,96] Osteoperiosteal flaps for transport of small and large alveolar segments have been popularized by Jensen.[97–101] The key to this procedure is to perform minimal reflection of the surrounding soft tissue in order to maintain adequate blood supply to the segment. The soft tissue cannot undergo excessive stretch which would embarrass blood supply.

Segmental Horizontal Deficiencies

Alveolar split osteotomy can be used to widen a horizontally deficient mandibular alveolus. To perform this technique, there must be at least 2 mm of crestal bone width. The procedure is performed through a minimally reflected crestal incision. Unlike the maxilla that readily expands, separate vertical and inferior osteotomies must be performed in the mandible to expand the alveolus because of the thick cortical plates. These osteotomies are usually performed with a piezoelectric drill through minimal tunneling.[54–56,58,102] With the use of sequentially expanding osteotomes, the bone can be forced buccally. Interposition (inlay) bone grafts with either banked or autogenous bone can be placed to keep the segments separated. If the segment is unstable, then a small miniplate can be placed for stabilization. Closure can be performed with or without a resorbable membrane.

Segmental Vertical Defects

Segmental vertical osteotomies are performed through a vestibular incision. A releasing incision is not needed. Soft tissue reflection is only enough to perform the osteotomy (**Fig. 8**). The osteotomy has both vertical and horizontal components. The horizontal component of the osteotomy is placed so that the strength of the basal bone is not significantly compromised and the transport segment is large enough for

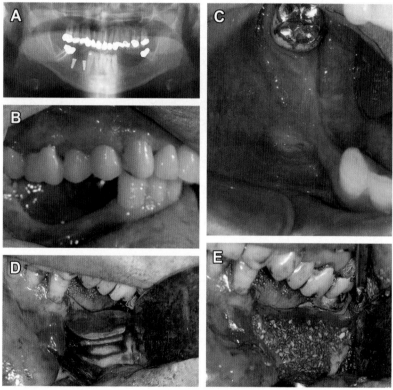

Fig. 8. Vascularized osteotomy for vertical augmentation of the mandible. (*A*) Preoperative panoramic radiograph of a patient with horizontal deficiency of the left posterior mandible. (*B*) Mirror view of the left posterior mandibular ridge (*lateral view*). (*C*) Mirror view of the left posterior mandibular ridge (*occlusal view*). (*D*) Mandibular osteotomy performed with interpositional bone graft. (*E*) Particulate bone graft has been packed around the osteotomy site. (*F*) Mirror view showing the site has been closed primarily. (*G*) Postoperative panoramic radiograph showing the reconstructed left mandibular ridge. (*H*) Panoramic radiograph with implants placed in the left mandible. (*I*) Mirror view of the restored left mandible (*lateral view*). (*J*) Mirror view of the restored left mandible (*occlusal view*). (*K*) Panoramic radiograph with restored implants in the left mandible. (Case provided by Kenneth J. Zouhary, DDS, MD, Chief of Oral & Maxillofacial Surgery, Birmingham VA Medical Center.)

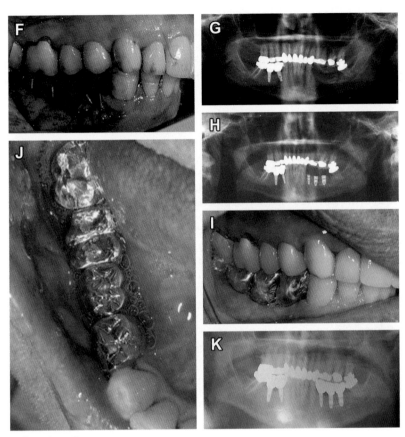

Fig. 8. (*continued*)

stabilization if needed. The vertical arms of the osteotomy connect the outer aspect of the horizontal osteotomy to the crest of the alveolus. There are usually two vertical arms, placed on either side of the planned alveolar segment that will be transported. The vertical arms should slightly converge toward the base of the transport segment. Once the bony cuts are made, the segment is moved to the desired level. Block or particulate inlay graft is used to hold the segment in the desired position. If particulate graft is used without a miniplate for stabilization, a mineralized bone graft material is preferable. If additional stability is needed, a miniplate can be placed. Since the incision is made in the vestibule, a single layered tension free closure is usually easily achieved.

Vertical Deficiency of the Mandibular Arch

Total mandibular osteotomy for correction of vertical deficiency of the mandible should be performed with caution. In cases of mandibular atrophy, an osteotomy may weaken the mandible and predispose it to fracture. Although absolute minimum height that must be present before considering this technique has not established, there must be enough bone to safely perform the osteotomy. The procedure is performed through a vestibular incision. Once the mental nerves have been identified and protected, the dissection is carried to the level of the planned osteotomy. Minimal periosteal reflection is performed. The planned osteotomy is performed with a piezo-electric drill, staying above the inferior alveolar nerve posterior to the mental foramen. Once the osteotomy is complete, the alveolar segment is moved superiorly to the desired height. The segment is stabilized with miniplates and interpositional bone graft. A tension-free closure can be performed with resorbable suture (eg, Vicryl or Monocryl).

POSTOPERATIVE CARE

Postoperative care for bone grafting treatment includes use of antibiotics such as amoxicillin or clindamycin for 7 to 10 days. Patients are placed on a chlorhexadine mouth rinse for at least the first 2 to 4 weeks. If a wound dehiscence develops, the patient is maintained on chlorhexadine mouth rinse until the second-stage surgery. If exposure of hardware occurs, appropriate cleaning should also include use of a soft toothbrush to remove any plaque or debris and irrigation. Follow-up visits are usually at 2 weeks, 1 month, and 3 months postoperatively. Temporization varies primarily based on if the patient is partially dentate. Most patients with some teeth can undergo immediate temporization using a partially or completely tooth-born prosthesis. Edentulous patients could undergo immediate temporization by relining an existing denture. However, to avoid pressure on the wound, in patients where hardware has been place, a period of rest is usually indicated to minimize the risk of wound dehiscence. The temporization could be delayed 2 to 4 weeks. In patients with atrophic mandibles that have undergone complete or segmental osteotomies, a strict non-chew diet for 6 to 8 weeks is recommended to minimize the risk of fracture. The

---

Box 1
Recommended options for defect reconstruction

I. Horizontal segmental defects

Onlay block graft with rigid membrane

Onlay particulate graft with membrane

Vascularized osteotomy with mineralized or block inlay graft

II. Horizontal deficiency of the entire arch

Onlay block graft with membrane

Onlay particulate graft with rigid membrane

Onlay particulate mineralized graft with membrane

Vascularized osteotomy with mineralized or block inlay graft

III. Vertical segmental defects

Onlay block graft with membrane

Onlay particulate graft with rigid membrane

Vascularized osteotomy with mineralized or block inlay graft

Vascularized osteotomy with inlay graft and rigid stabilization

IV. Vertical deficiency of the entire arch

Onlay block graft with membrane

Onlay particulate graft with rigid membrane

Vascularized osteotomy with inlay graft and rigid stabilization

second-stage surgery should be planned for 4 to 6 months postoperatively. The hardware is usually removed at second-stage surgery when implants are placed.

DISCUSSION

Determination of what technique should be used when reconstructing a segmental defect of the mandible or an entire arch is largely surgeon preference; however, there are some situations where one technique would have greater success (**Box 1**).

Vertical augmentation can be particularly difficult to reconstruct due to soft tissue collapse over the graft if the space is not maintained. When performing vertical ridge augmentation, it is important to maintain the space with a block graft protected with a membrane, particulate graft protected with a rigid membrane, or the use of an osteomucoperiosteal flap.[9,45,78,79,83,99–101,103–106]

Although autogenous bone has been considered the gold standard in the past, more recent studies have shown that vertical and horizontal augmentation can be successfully performed with allogeneic and xenogenic grafts when properly protected with the appropriate membrane.[61,62,64,67,82,83,107,108] The use of growth factors can enhance the success of grafts.[109–112]

REFERENCES

1. Gerry RG. Alveolar ridge reconstruction with osseous autograft: report of case. J Oral Surg (Chic) 1956;14(1):74–8.
2. Aghaloo TL, Moy PK. Which hard tissue augmentation techniques are the most successful in furnishing bony support for implant placement? Int J Oral Maxillofac Implants 2007;22:49–70.
3. Amrani S, Anastassov GE, Montazem AH. Mandibular ramus/coronoid process grafts in maxillofacial reconstructive surgery. J Oral Maxillofac Surg 2010;68(3): 641–6.
4. Esposito M, Grusovin MG, Felice P, et al. The efficacy of horizontal and vertical bone augmentation procedures for dental implants—a Cochrane systematic review. Eur J Oral Implantol 2009;2(3):167–84.
5. Gutta R, Waite PD. Cranial bone grafting and simultaneous implants: a submental technique to reconstruct the atrophic mandible. Br J Oral Maxillofac Surg 2008;46(6):477–9.
6. Hopkins R. A sandwich mandibular osteotomy: a preliminary report. Br J Oral Surg 1982;20(3):155–67.
7. Aalam AA, Nowzari H. Mandibular cortical bone grafts part 1: anatomy, healing process, and influencing factors. Compend Contin Educ Dent 2007;28(4): 206–12 [quiz: 13].
8. Donovan MG, Dickerson NC, Mitchell JC. Calvarial bone harvest and grafting techniques for maxillary and mandibular implant surgery. Atlas Oral Maxillofac Surg Clin North Am 1994;2(2):109–22.
9. Pikos MA. Atrophic posterior maxilla and mandible: alveolar ridge reconstruction with mandibular block autografts. Alpha Omegan 2005;98(3):34–45.
10. Pikos MA. Mandibular block autografts for alveolar ridge augmentation. Atlas Oral Maxillofac Surg Clin North Am 2005;13(2):91–107.
11. Pikos MA. Block autografts for localized ridge augmentation: part II. The posterior mandible. Implant Dent 2000;9(1):67–75.
12. Boyne PJ. Autogenous cancellous bone and marrow transplants. Clin Orthop Relat Res 1970;73:199–209.

13. Cushing M. Autogenous red marrow grafts: their potential for induction of osteo-genesis. J Periodontol 1969;40(8):492–7.
14. Dragoo MR, Sullivan HC. A clinical and histological evaluation of autogenous iliac bone grafts in humans. I. Wound healing 2 to 8 months. J Periodontol 1973;44(10):599–613.
15. Rivault AF, Toto PD, Levy S, et al. Autogenous bone grafts: osseous coagulum and osseous retrograde procedures in primates. J Periodontol 1971;42(12): 787–96.
16. Buchman SR, Ozaki W. The ultrastructure and resorptive pattern of cancellous onlay bone grafts in the craniofacial skeleton. Ann Plast Surg 1999;43(1): 49–56.
17. Ozaki W, Buchman SR. Volume maintenance of onlay bone grafts in the cranio-facial skeleton: microarchitecture versus embryologic origin. Plast Reconstr Surg 1998;102(2):291–9.
18. Ozaki W, Buchman SR, Goldstein SA, et al. A comparative analysis of the micro-architecture of cortical membranous and cortical endochondral onlay bone grafts in the craniofacial skeleton. Plast Reconstr Surg 1999;104(1):139–47.
19. Zins JE, Whitaker LA. Membranous versus endochondral bone: implications for craniofacial reconstruction. Plast Reconstr Surg 1983;72(6):778–85.
20. Zins JE, Whitaker LA. Membranous vs endochondral bone autografts: implica-tions for craniofacial reconstruction. Surg Forum 1979;30:521–3.
21. Clavero J, Lundgren S. Ramus or chin grafts for maxillary sinus inlay and local onlay augmentation: comparison of donor site morbidity and complications. Clin Implant Dent Relat Res 2003;5(3):154–60.
22. Felice P, Iezzi G, Lizio G, et al. Reconstruction of atrophied posterior mandible with inlay technique and mandibular ramus block graft for implant prosthetic rehabilitation. J Oral Maxillofac Surg 2009;67(2):372–80.
23. Hoppenreijs TJ, Nijdam ES, Freihofer HP. The chin as a donor site in early secondary osteoplasty: a retrospective clinical and radiological evaluation. J Craniomaxillofac Surg 1992;20(3):119–24.
24. Precious DS, Smith WP. The use of mandibular symphyseal bone in maxillofacial surgery. Br J Oral Maxillofac Surg 1992;30(3):148–52.
25. Booij A, Raghoebar GM, Jansma J, et al. Morbidity of chin bone transplants used for reconstructing alveolar defects in cleft patients. Cleft Palate Craniofac J 2005;42(5):533–8.
26. Park HD, Min CK, Kwak HH, et al. Topography of the outer mandibular symphy-seal region with reference to the autogenous bone graft. Int J Oral Maxillofac Surg 2004;33(8):781–5.
27. Chiapasco M, Abati S, Romeo E, et al. Clinical outcome of autogenous bone blocks or guided bone regeneration with e-PTFE membranes for the reconstruc-tion of narrow edentulous ridges. Clin Oral Implants Res 1999;10(4):278–88.
28. Gellrich NC, Held U, Schoen R, et al. Alveolar zygomatic buttress: a new donor site for limited preimplant augmentation procedures. J Oral Maxillofac Surg 2007;65(2):275–80.
29. Drew H, Zweig B. Use of a buccal exostosis autograft for alveolar ridge augmen-tation: an aid to implant placement. J N J Dent Assoc 2007;78(3):40–2.
30. Tolstunov L. Maxillary tuberosity block bone graft: innovative technique and case report. J Oral Maxillofac Surg 2009;67(8):1723–9.
31. Moraes Junior EF, Damante CA, Araujo SR. Torus palatinus: a graft option for alveolar ridge reconstruction. Int J Periodontics Restorative Dent 2010;30(3): 283–9.

32. Diaz-Romeral-Bautista M, Manchon-Miralles A, Asenjo-Cabezon J, et al. Autogenous calvarium bone grafting as a treatment for severe bone resorption in the upper maxilla: a case report. Med Oral Patol Oral Cir Bucal 2010;15(2):e361–5.
33. Gutta R, Waite PD. Outcomes of calvarial bone grafting for alveolar ridge reconstruction. Int J Oral Maxillofac Implants 2009;24(1):131–6.
34. Cranin AN, Demirdjan E, DiGregorio R. A comparison of allogeneic and autogenous iliac monocortical grafts to augment the deficient alveolar ridge in a canine model. I. Clinical study. J Oral Implantol 2003;29(3):124–31.
35. Crespi R, Vinci R, Cappare P, et al. Calvarial versus iliac crest for autologous bone graft material for a sinus lift procedure: a histomorphometric study. Int J Oral Maxillofac Implants 2007;22(4):527–32.
36. Felice P, Marchetti C, Iezzi G, et al. Vertical ridge augmentation of the atrophic posterior mandible with interpositional bloc grafts: bone from the iliac crest vs. bovine anorganic bone. Clinical and histological results up to one year after loading from a randomized–controlled clinical trial. Clin Oral Implants Res 2009;20(12):1386–93.
37. Bogdan S, Nemeth Z, Huszar T, et al. The proximal tibia. A possible donor site in preprosthetic surgery. Fogorv Sz 2008;101(2):58–63.
38. Bogdan S, Nemeth Z, Huszar T, et al. Comparison of postoperative complications following bone harvesting from two different donor sites for autologous bone replacement (hip bone and proximal epiphysis of the tibia). Orv Hetil 2009;150(7):305–11.
39. Catone GA, Reimer BL, McNeir D, et al. Tibial autogenous cancellous bone as an alternative donor site in maxillofacial surgery: a preliminary report. J Oral Maxillofac Surg 1992;50(12):1258–63.
40. Marchena JM, Block MS, Stover JD. Tibial bone harvesting under intravenous sedation: morbidity and patient experiences. J Oral Maxillofac Surg 2002;60(10):1151–4.
41. O'Keeffe RM Jr, Riemer BL, Butterfield SL. Harvesting of autogenous cancellous bone graft from the proximal tibial metaphysis. A review of 230 cases. J Orthop Trauma 1991;5(4):469–74.
42. Pensler J, McCarthy JG. The calvarial donor site: an anatomic study in cadavers. Plast Reconstr Surg 1985;75(5):648–51.
43. Moreira-Gonzalez A, Papay FE, Zins JE. Calvarial thickness and its relation to cranial bone harvest. Plast Reconstr Surg 2006;117(6):1964–71.
44. Al-Sebaei MO, Papageorge MB, Woo T. Technique for in-office cranial bone harvesting. J Oral Maxillofac Surg 2004;62:120–2.
45. Salvato G, Agliardi E. Calvarial bone grafts in severe maxillary atrophy: preprosthetic surgery with sedation. Implant Dent 2007;16(4):356–61.
46. Iturriaga MT, Ruiz CC. Maxillary sinus reconstruction with calvarium bone grafts and endosseous implants. J Oral Maxillofac Surg 2004;62(3):344–7.
47. Kao SY, Yeung TC, Chou IC, et al. Reconstruction of the severely resorbed atrophic edentulous ridge of the maxilla and mandible for implant rehabilitation: report of a case. J Oral Implantol 2002;28(3):128–32.
48. Marx RE. Bone harvest from the posterior ilium. Atlas Oral Maxillofac Surg Clin North Am 2005;13(2):109–18.
49. Marx RE, Morales MJ. Morbidity from bone harvest in major jaw reconstruction: a randomized trial comparing the lateral anterior and posterior approaches to the ilium. J Oral Maxillofac Surg 1988;46(3):196–203.
50. Beirne OR. Comparison of complications after bone removal from lateral and medial plates of the anterior ilium for mandibular augmentation. Int J Oral Maxillofac Surg 1986;15(3):269–72.

51. Falkensammer N, Kirmeier R, Arnetzl C, et al. Modified iliac bone harvesting—morbidity and patients' experience. J Oral Maxillofac Surg 2009;67(8):1700–5.

52. Nkenke E, Weisbach V, Winckler E, et al. Morbidity of harvesting of bone grafts from the iliac crest for preprosthetic augmentation procedures: a prospective study. Int J Oral Maxillofac Surg 2004;33(2):157–63.

53. Schaaf H, Lendeckel S, Howaldt HP, et al. Donor site morbidity after bone harvesting from the anterior iliac crest. Oral Surg Oral Med Oral Pathol Oral Radiol Endod 2010;109(1):52–8.

54. Dibart S, Sebaoun JD, Surmenian J. Piezocision: a minimally invasive, periodontally accelerated orthodontic tooth movement procedure. Compend Contin Educ Dent 2009;30(6):342–4, 346, 348–50.

55. Sohn DS, Lee JS, An KM, et al. Piezoelectric internal sinus elevation (PISE) technique: a new method for internal sinus elevation. Implant Dent 2009;18(6):458–63.

56. Lee HJ, Ahn MR, Sohn DS. Piezoelectric distraction osteogenesis in the atrophic maxillary anterior area: a case report. Implant Dent 2007;16(3):227–34.

57. Moon JW, Choi BJ, Lee WH, et al. Reconstruction of atrophic anterior mandible using piezoelectric sandwich osteotomy: a case report. Implant Dent 2009;18(3):195–202.

58. Sohn DS, Ahn MR, Lee WH, et al. Piezoelectric osteotomy for intraoral harvesting of bone blocks. Int J Periodontics Restorative Dent 2007;27(2):127–31.

59. Quereshy FA, Dhaliwal HS, El SA, et al. Resorbable screw fixation for cortical onlay bone grafting: a pilot study with preliminary results. J Oral Maxillofac Surg 2010;68(10):2497–502.

60. Burger BW. Use of ultrasound-activated resorbable poly-D-L-lactide pins (SonicPins) and foil panels (Resorb-X) for horizontal bone augmentation of the maxillary and mandibular alveolar ridges. J Oral Maxillofac Surg 2010;68(7):1656–61.

61. Barone A, Varanini P, Orlando B, et al. Deep-frozen allogeneic onlay bone grafts for reconstruction of atrophic maxillary alveolar ridges: a preliminary study. J Oral Maxillofac Surg 2009;67(6):1300–6.

62. Dori S, Peleg M, Barnea E. Alveolar ridge augmentation with hip corticocancellous allogenic block graft prior to implant placement. Refuat Hapeh Vehashinayim 2008;25(3):28–38, 54.

63. Petrungaro PS, Amar S. Localized ridge augmentation with allogenic block grafts prior to implant placement: case reports and histologic evaluations. Implant Dent 2005;14(2):139–48.

64. Waasdorp J, Reynolds MA. Allogeneic bone onlay grafts for alveolar ridge augmentation: a systematic review. Int J Oral Maxillofac Implants 2010;25(3):525–31.

65. Askari A, Amato F, Abitbol T. The regenerative potential of ePTFE membranes and freeze-dried bone allografts—two case reports. Periodontal Clin Investig 1994;16(2):20–4.

66. Becker W, Hujoel P, Becker BE. Effect of barrier membranes and autologous bone grafts on ridge width preservation around implants. Clin Implant Dent Relat Res 2002;4(3):143–9.

67. Beitlitum I, Artzi Z, Nemcovsky CE. Clinical evaluation of particulate allogeneic with and without autogenous bone grafts and resorbable collagen membranes for bone augmentation of atrophic alveolar ridges. Clin Oral Implants Res 2010;21(11):1242–50.

68. Chen CC, Wang HL, Smith F, et al. Evaluation of a collagen membrane with and without bone grafts in treating periodontal intrabony defects. J Periodontol 1995;66(10):838–47.

69. Chiapasco M, Zaniboni M. Clinical outcomes of GBR procedures to correct peri-implant dehiscences and fenestrations: a systematic review. Clin Oral Implants Res 2009;20(Suppl 4):113–23.
70. Fugazzotto PA. GBR using bovine bone matrix and resorbable and nonresorbable membranes. Part 1: histologic results. Int J Periodontics Restorative Dent 2003;23(4):361–9.
71. Gielkens PF, Bos RR, Raghoebar GM, et al. Is there evidence that barrier membranes prevent bone resorption in autologous bone grafts during the healing period? A systematic review. Int J Oral Maxillofac Implants 2007;22(3): 390–8.
72. Gielkens PF, Schortinghuis J, de Jong JR, et al. The influence of barrier membranes on autologous bone grafts. J Dent Res 2008;87(11):1048–52.
73. Hammerle CH, Jung RE, Yaman D, et al. Ridge augmentation by applying bioresorbable membranes and deproteinized bovine bone mineral: a report of twelve consecutive cases. Clin Oral Implants Res 2008;19(1):19–25.
74. Rasmusson L, Meredith N, Kahnberg KE, et al. Effects of barrier membranes on bone resorption and implant stability in onlay bone grafts. An experimental study. Clin Oral Implants Res 1999;10(4):267–77.
75. Stavropoulos F, Dahlin C, Ruskin JD, et al. A comparative study of barrier membranes as graft protectors in the treatment of localized bone defects. An experimental study in a canine model. Clin Oral Implants Res 2004;15(4): 435–42.
76. Cordaro L, Amade DS, Cordaro M. Clinical results of alveolar ridge augmentation with mandibular block bone grafts in partially edentulous patients prior to implant placement. Clin Oral Implants Res 2002;13(1):103–11.
77. Gutta R, Baker RA, Bartolucci AA, et al. Barrier membranes used for ridge augmentation: is there an optimal pore size? J Oral Maxillofac Surg 2009; 67(6):1218–25.
78. Louis PJ, Gutta R, Said-Al-Naief N, et al. Reconstruction of the maxilla and mandible with particulate bone graft and titanium mesh for implant placement. J Oral Maxillofac Surg 2008;66(2):235–45.
79. von Arx T, Hardt N, Wallkamm B. The TIME technique: a new method for localized alveolar ridge augmentation prior to placement of dental implants. Int J Oral Maxillofac Implants 1996;11(3):387–94.
80. von Arx T, Hardt N, Wallkamm B. The TIME technic. Local osteoplasty with micro-titanium mesh (TIME) for alveolar ridge augmentation. Schweiz Monatsschr Zahnmed 1995;105(5):650–63.
81. von Arx T, Kurt B. Implant placement and simultaneous periimplant bone grafting using a microtitanium mesh for graft stabilization. Int J Periodontics Restorative Dent 1998;18(2):117–27.
82. Torres J, Tamimi F, Alkhraisat MH, et al. Platelet-rich plasma may prevent titanium–mesh exposure in alveolar ridge augmentation with anorganic bovine bone. J Clin Periodontol 2010;37(10):943–51.
83. Artzi Z, Dayan D, Alpern Y, et al. Vertical ridge augmentation using xenogenic material supported by a configured titanium mesh: clinicohistopathologic and histochemical study. Int J Oral Maxillofac Implants 2003;18(3):440–6.
84. Bosker H, van Dijk L. The transmandibular implant: a 12-year follow-up study. J Oral Maxillofac Surg 1989;47(5):442–50.
85. Bosker H, Wardle ML. Muscular reconstruction to improve the deterioration of facial appearance and speech caused by mandibular atrophy: technique and case reports. Br J Oral Maxillofac Surg 1999;37(4):277–84.

86. Byrne RP, Hinds EC. The ramus "C" osteotomy with body sagittal split. J Oral Surg 1974;32(4):259–63.

87. Dupont C, Ciaburro TH, Prevost Y. Simplifying the Le Fort I type of maxillary osteotomy. Plast Reconstr Surg 1974;54(2):142–7.

88. Freihofer HP Jr. The lip profile after correction of retromaxillism in cleft and non-cleft patients. J Maxillofac Surg 1976;4(3):136–41.

89. Steinhauser EW. Advancement of the mandible by sagittal ramus split and suprahyoid myotomy. J Oral Surg 1973;31(7):516–21.

90. Steinhauser EW. Variations of Le Fort II osteotomies for correction of midfacial deformities. J Maxillofac Surg 1980;8(4):258–65.

91. Tessier P. Treatment of facial dysmorphias in craniofacial dysostosis, Crouzon's and Apert's diseases. Total osteotomy and sagittal displacement of the facial massive. Faciostenosis, sequelae of Lefort 3 fracture. Dtsch Zahn Mund Kieferheilkd Zentralbl Gesamte 1971;57(9):302–20.

92. Bell WH. Revascularization and bone healing after anterior maxillary osteotomy: a study using adult rhesus monkeys. J Oral Surg 1969;27(4):249–55.

93. Bell WH, Fonseca RJ, Kenneky JW, et al. Bone healing and revascularization after total maxillary osteotomy. J Oral Surg 1975;33(4):253–60.

94. Bell WH, Levy BM. Revascularization and bone healing after maxillary corticotomies. J Oral Surg 1972;30(9):640–8.

95. Bell WH, Schendel SA, Finn RA. Revascularization after surgical repositioning of one-tooth dento-osseous segments. J Oral Surg 1978;36(10):757–65.

96. Quejada JG, Kawamura H, Finn RA, et al. Wound healing associated with segmental total maxillary osteotomy. J Oral Maxillofac Surg 1986;44(5): 366–77.

97. Jensen OT. Alveolar segmental sandwich osteotomies for posterior edentulous mandibular sites for dental implants. J Oral Maxillofac Surg 2006;64(3):471–5.

98. Jensen OT. Distraction osteogenesis and its use with dental implants. Dent Implantol Update 1999;10(5):33–6.

99. Jensen OT, Bell W, Cottam J. Osteoperiosteal flaps and local osteotomies for alveolar reconstruction. Oral Maxillofac Surg Clin North Am 2010;22(3): 331–46, vi.

100. Jensen OT, Kuhlke L, Bedard JF, et al. Alveolar segmental sandwich osteotomy for anterior maxillary vertical augmentation prior to implant placement. J Oral Maxillofac Surg 2006;64(2):290–6.

101. Jensen OT, Mogyoros R, Owen Z, et al. Island osteoperiosteal flap for alveolar bone reconstruction. J Oral Maxillofac Surg 2010;68(3):539–46.

102. Peivandi A, Bugnet R, Debize E, et al. Piezoelectric osteotomy: applications in periodontal and implant surgery. Rev Stomatol Chir Maxillofac 2007;108(5): 431–40.

103. Maestre-Ferrin L, Boronat-Lopez A, Penarrocha-Diago M. Augmentation procedures for deficient edentulous ridges, using onlay autologous grafts: an update. Med Oral Patol Oral Cir Bucal 2009;14(8):e402–7.

104. Gongloff RK, Cole M, Whitlow W, et al. Titanium mesh and particulate cancellous bone and marrow grafts to augment the maxillary alveolar ridge. Int J Oral Maxillofac Surg 1986;15(3):263–8.

105. Roccuzzo M, Ramieri G, Spada MC, et al. Vertical alveolar ridge augmentation by means of a titanium mesh and autogenous bone grafts. Clin Oral Implants Res 2004;15(1):73–81.

106. Aparicio C, Jensen OT. Alveolar ridge widening by distraction osteogenesis: a case report. Pract Proced Aesthet Dent 2001;13(8):663–8 [quiz: 70].

107. Fontana F, Santoro F, Maiorana C, et al. Clinical and histologic evaluation of allogeneic bone matrix versus autogenous bone chips associated with titanium-reinforced e-PTFE membrane for vertical ridge augmentation: a prospective pilot study. Int J Oral Maxillofac Implants 2008;23(6):1003–12.
108. Pieri F, Corinaldesi G, Fini M, et al. Alveolar ridge augmentation with titanium mesh and a combination of autogenous bone and anorganic bovine bone: a 2-year prospective study. J Periodontol 2008;79(11):2093–103.
109. Jung RE, Thoma DS, Hammerle CH. Assessment of the potential of growth factors for localized alveolar ridge augmentation: a systematic review. J Clin Periodontol 2008;35(Suppl 8):255–81.
110. Herford AS, Boyne PJ, Williams RP. Clinical applications of rhBMP-2 in maxillofacial surgery. J Calif Dent Assoc 2007;35(5):335–41.
111. Zhang H, Zhou X, Wang X. Mandibular ridge augmentation by sandwich osteotomy and BMP-HA implantation. Zhonghua Kou Qiang Yi Xue Za Zhi 1997;32(1):37–9.
112. Jung RE, Windisch SI, Eggenschwiler AM, et al. A randomized–controlled clinical trial evaluating clinical and radiological outcomes after 3 and 5 years of dental implants placed in bone regenerated by means of GBR techniques with or without the addition of BMP-2. Clin Oral Implants Res 2009;20(7):660–6.
113. Montazem A, Valauri DV, St-Hilaire H, et al. The mandibular symphysis as a donor site in maxillofacial bone grafting: a quantitative anatomic study. J Oral Maxillofac Surg 2000;58(12):1368–71.
114. Gungormus M, Yilmaz AB, Ertas U, et al. Evaluation of the mandible as an alternative autogenous bone source for oral and maxillofacial reconstruction. J Int Med Res 2002;30(3):260–4.
115. Gungormus M, Yavuz MS. The ascending ramus of the mandible as a donor site in maxillofacial bone grafting. J Oral Maxillofac Surg 2002;60(11):1316–8.
116. Li KK, Schwartz HC. Mandibular body bone in facial plastic and reconstructive surgery. Laryngoscope 1996;106(4):504–6.
117. Choung PH, Kim SG. The coronoid process for paranasal augmentation in the correction of midfacial concavity. Oral Surg Oral Med Oral Pathol Oral Radiol Endod 2001;91(1):28–33.

Maxillary Autogenous Bone Grafting

Craig M. Misch, DDS, MDS[a,b],*

KEYWORDS

• Maxilla • Autogenous • Bone grafting • Dental implants

Reconstruction of the atrophic maxilla for dental implant placement has many unique considerations (**Figs. 1–20**). After tooth extraction, the greatest loss of bone in the maxilla occurs facially. Horizontal bone resorption can approach 50% of the ridge width at 12 months.[1] The use of a soft tissue borne–prosthesis causes continued medial resorption and loss of vertical bone height.[2] As a result, the atrophic residual ridge may be significantly palatal to the prosthetic tooth position. Efforts to reconstruct the atrophic maxilla to its original form usually require buccal bone augmentation. The surgeon must also contend with the maxillary sinuses and nasal cavity as anatomic limitations that may need bone grafting. The maxillary bone is often less dense than the mandible, especially in the posterior regions below the sinuses.[3] Aesthetic zone reconstruction in the partially edentulous anterior maxilla can be especially challenging when a high lip line exposes gingiva.

There are several methods available to augment the atrophic maxilla, including onlay bone grafting, sinus/nasal bone grafting, guided bone regeneration, interpositional grafting, ridge splitting, and distraction osteogenesis. The choice of a particular technique depends on the need for horizontal or vertical augmentation, degree of atrophy, type of prosthesis, and clinician or patient preference. Autogenous bone grafting offers a well-proven predictable method for ridge augmentation and defect repair for dental implant placement. There are several advantages to using autogenous bone grafts.[4] Autogenous block bone grafts have a shorter healing period than other approaches such as guided bone regeneration using bone substitutes. This graft usually requires only 4 months of healing before implants may be inserted. On incorporation, the quality of the graft often exceeds the density of the native maxillary bone. This enhanced quality improves implant stability and can shorten healing time. The

This article was previously published in the May 2011 issue of *Oral and Maxillofacial Surgery Clinics of North America*.

[a] Private Practice, Oral & Maxillofacial Surgery and Prosthodontics, 120 Tuttle Avenue, Sarasota, FL 34237, USA

[b] Department of Implant Dentistry, New York University College of Dentistry, 345 East 24th Street, New York, NY 10010, USA

* Private Practice, Oral & Maxillofacial Surgery and Prosthodontics, 120 Tuttle Avenue, Sarasota, FL 34237.

E-mail address: misch@bonegraft.com

dental.theclinics.com

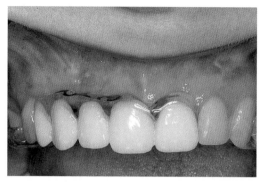

Fig. 1. Traumatic avulsion of maxillary teeth and resulting defect. A CT scan template is fabricated with barium teeth to reveal the planned tooth position.

cost of autogenous bone is obviously much less than using bone substitutes, membranes, and/or recombinant growth factors. Block bone grafts may be preferred to osteotomy techniques (ridge splitting, interpositional grafts) because they can 3-dimensionally reconstruct the lost anatomic ridge contour. Autogenous bone grafts have proven to be most effective in managing larger bone defects. Although sinus bone grafting may not require the routine use of autogenous bone, autogenous bone use may be beneficial when treating large pneumatized sinuses with minimal remaining bone.[5] This article primarily focuses on the use of autogenous onlay bone grafts to reconstruct the atrophic maxilla.

PROSTHETIC TREATMENT PLANNING

It is important to define the prosthetic goals before the maxillary reconstruction. The design of the final prosthesis determines the number of implants required and the ideal

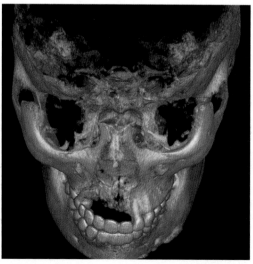

Fig. 2. A 3-dimensional view of the CT scan of maxillary teeth with the barium template, revealing the maxillary defect and augmentation requirements.

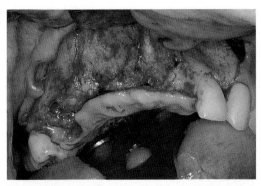

Fig. 3. Maxillary defect with horizontal and vertical bone deficiencies.

positions of implants. If there is inadequate available bone for implant placement in the desired locations, then bone augmentation is considered. This concept has been termed prosthetic guided bone augmentation. Computed tomography (CT) is extremely useful in assessing the ridge deficiency and volume of bone augmentation required.[6] Radiographic templates allow the clinician to evaluate the ideal prosthetic tooth position in relationship to the atrophic ridge.[7] In addition, an implant planning software can be used with the scan to precisely evaluate the reconstructive needs of the patient.[8] It is difficult to provide absolute guidelines for the number and distribution of implants to support a particular type of prosthesis. However, generalizations may be made based on biomechanical support, long-term studies, and clinical experience. When only the minimum number of implants are used, the prosthesis may be at risk if complications occur. The philosophy of "protect the prosthesis" is a prudent guideline in treatment planning and design of the implant support system.[9]

The planning for posterior implant support in the edentulous maxilla has been simplified with sinus bone grafting techniques and zygoma implants.[10,11] The residual ridge anterior to the sinuses is therefore the key region to evaluate for implant placement. From a prosthetic perspective, anterior abutments are necessary for proper load distribution and mechanical support. Ignoring the atrophic anterior maxilla and only placing posterior implants can have undesirable prosthetic consequences. One must keep in mind that the maxilla resorbs medially such that the residual ridge is palatal to the position of the teeth. Functional use of the anterior teeth, for incising

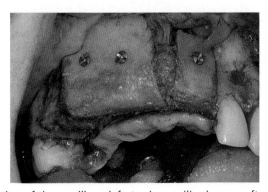

Fig. 4. Reconstruction of the maxillary defect using an iliac bone graft.

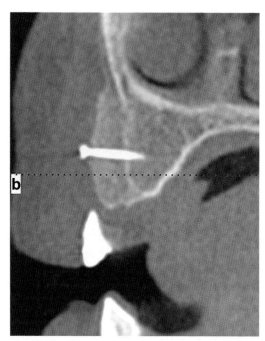

Fig. 5. A CT scan of the healed graft, showing minimal resorption and favorable bone volume for implant placement.

and anterior guidance, can cause a tripping action on an upper overdenture. A continuous connecting bar across the anterior maxilla acts as a vertical stop to resist overdenture displacement. A lack of anterior abutments for a fixed prosthesis creates a cantilever effect that can lead to complications such as screw loosening, screw breakage, marginal bone loss, and implant fracture.[12–15] These problems are magnified in patients with biomechanical risk factors such as strong masticatory dynamics, parafunctional habits, or opposing natural dentition/fixed implant prosthesis.[16–18] Therefore, when the residual ridge is deficient in the anterior maxilla, autogenous block

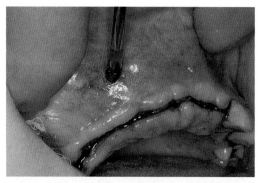

Fig. 6. Removal of the fixation screws through a mucosal incision for implant placement after a 4-month healing period.

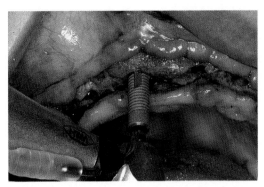

Fig. 7. Placement of the implants into the incorporated bone graft.

bone grafts can be used to predictably develop sites for implant placement. This site development using implants is accomplished in a staged manner with implant placement following graft incorporation.

EDENTULOUS MAXILLA
Implant-Supported Overdenture

Clinical studies have found that implant failure rates are often significantly higher for maxillary overdentures than any other type of implant prosthesis.[19,20] This higher failure rate may be because of less bone volume and poorer bone quality as well implant distribution, prosthetic design, and opposing occlusion. Although the use of 2 implants for overdenture support is a well-documented option in the mandible, this approach is less recommended in the maxilla.[21] Many patients with minimal atrophy of the upper jaw are able to tolerate a maxillary complete denture. It is not until the maxilla becomes more resorbed that the patient experiences problems with stability and retention of the prosthesis. With increased atrophy, there is less available bone for implant placement and less residual ridge for prosthetic support. Higher loads are placed on 2 independent implants in soft-quality bone.[22] Studies have found higher implant failure rates and greater levels of marginal bone loss around independent maxillary implants supporting overdenture prostheses.[20,23–25] Although the cost is higher, the mechanical advantage of implant splinting with a connecting bar is preferred.[26]

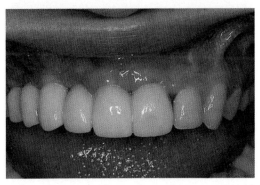

Fig. 8. Provisional tooth replacement using an immediate provisional bridge.

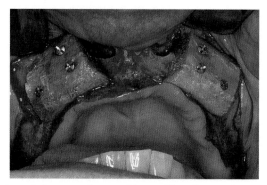

Fig. 9. Reconstruction of the severely atrophic maxilla using corticocancellous block bone grafts.

The minimum number of implants for support of a maxillary overdenture is 4. Two implants are typically positioned on each side of the maxilla anterior to the maxillary sinuses. The midline area is usually avoided to provide space for positioning denture teeth, minimize bulky palatal contours, and allow placement of anterior prosthetic attachments. The 4 implants should be splinted with a connecting bar.[9,25] This splinting requires preoperative planning in cases with less atrophy because greater interarch space is needed. The palate and posterior areas of the maxillary ridge may be used for additional prosthetic support.

A maxillary overdenture with 6 implants may be removable yet completely implant supported. Sinus bone grafting is often required to place the 2 additional posterior implants. As previously mentioned, avoiding implant placement in the midline area is preferred. Reduction of palatal coverage is a desired benefit of additional implant support. The 6 implants are cross-arch splinted with a connecting bar. Although 2 separate connecting bars have been proposed, this design is mechanically unfavorable because the overdenture has a tendency to rock from the lack of anterior support.[27]

Fixed Implant Prosthesis

The minimum number of implants proposed for support of a maxillary fixed prosthesis is 4. Although the early Swedish literature documented maxillary cases with as few as

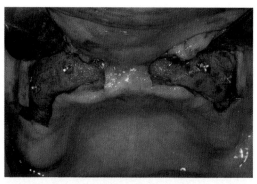

Fig. 10. Well-incorporated bone graft for implant placement after a 4-month healing period.

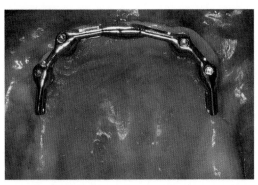

Fig. 11. Splinting of the 4 maxillary implants for support of an overdenture using an implant connecting bar.

4 implants, they more often recommended 6 placed anterior to the maxillary sinuses.[28] A higher failure rate was noted when only 4 implants were used.[29] More recently, the All-on-Four concept was introduced for treatment of the edentulous maxilla using 4 implants for a fixed prosthesis.[30] In this approach, the posterior implants are placed in a tilted manner to follow the anterior sinus border, extending the distal position of the implants. Although early results have been favorable, the obvious significant disadvantage is that loss of one implant will result in complete prosthetic failure. A more prudent approach is to consider a minimum of 6 implants for a maxillary fixed prosthesis. Implants should be evenly distributed across the maxilla, avoiding long pontic spans. Sinus bone grafting may be required to place the posterior implants. Greater numbers of implants (7–12) are recommended when mechanical risk factors are higher, bone volume is compromised, and/or bone density is poor.[9] Bone augmentation is often required in the atrophic maxilla, including sinus and/or onlay grafting, to provide the preferred number and distribution of implants. A greater number of implants (>6) are also advised when immediate loading with a fixed prosthesis is planned.[31]

The Aesthetic Zone

Bone remodeling following tooth loss can have a significant effect on the ability to properly place dental implants in the aesthetic zone. When the anterior maxilla is

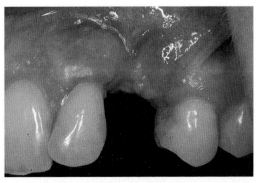

Fig. 12. Preoperative view of an alveolar defect after a failed attempt at repair using guided bone regeneration techniques.

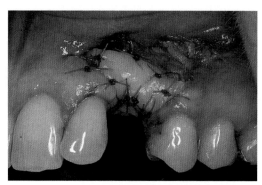

Fig. 13. Repairing the soft tissue defect before bone graft surgery using a gingival graft from the palate.

planned for grafting, an aesthetic zone evaluation is necessary. The surgeon should plan on providing adequate bone volume for implant placement as well as a proper soft tissue profile for the implant restoration. The amount of tooth and gingival exposure with a high smile is accessed. The need for lip support is evaluated when multiple teeth are missing. A diagnostic wax up helps determine the ideal tooth length and need for vertical augmentation to develop the proper tooth size. If the upper lip covers the defect, it may be an option to prosthetically replace the missing hard and soft tissues with gingival colored porcelain.

The soft tissue in the graft recipient site should be evaluated, including the amount of keratinized tissue and gingival biotype. It is often better to plan the correction of soft tissue problems before bone grafting. This correction will help reduce soft tissue complications (ie, wound dehiscence) and improve graft incorporation. Autogenous free gingival grafts from the palate may be used to increase the amount of keratinized tissue. Connective tissue grafts from the palate can be used to enhance mucosal thickness and improve graft coverage. Soft tissue corrective surgery must be performed at least 8 weeks before bone grafting. The surgeon should be aware that facial flap advancement over a bone graft moves the mucogingival junction palatally.

When failed maxillary incisors have significant facial bone loss, the osseous repair is usually not performed at the time of extraction. The normal gingival anatomy is disrupted by the flap advancement over the socket because primary soft tissue closure is

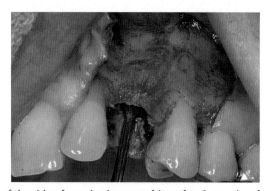

Fig. 14. Exposure of the ridge for onlay bone grafting after 2 months of soft tissue grafting.

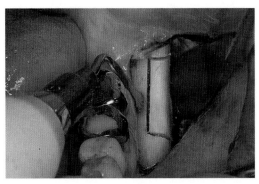

Fig. 15. Harvesting a cortical bone graft from the mandibular ramus using a piezoelectric saw.

necessary for bone grafting or membrane repair. The reconstruction of the alveolar defect is performed approximately 6 to 8 weeks after extraction to allow epithelialization over the socket, which allows the surgeon to perform the bone graft and adapt the flaps to maintain the soft tissue architecture.

The teeth adjacent to the graft site should also be evaluated before grafting. It is often preferred to extract compromised teeth before the bone graft surgery and allow the soft tissue to heal over the site. The marginal bone height on the teeth bordering the ridge defect determines the level that may be achieved with vertical bone augmentation. In some cases, it may be preferred to remove teeth with marginal bone loss to improve the ability to reconstruct the ridge.

BONE GRAFT DONOR SITES

Onlay bone grafts can be used to increase horizontal ridge width and/or vertical ridge height. The degree of jaw atrophy and amount of bone augmentation required for implant placement determines the preferred donor site for graft harvest. For the management of moderate ridge atrophy, bone grafts can be procured from intraoral donor sites, such as the symphysis and ramus of the mandible. These donor sites are desirable because the surgery may be performed in the office. Intraoral bone grafts are primarily cortical and used for veneer grafting narrow ridges or modest vertical augmentation.

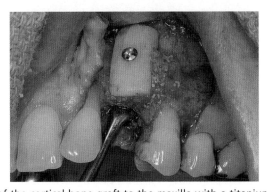

Fig. 16. Fixation of the cortical bone graft to the maxilla with a titanium alloy lag screw.

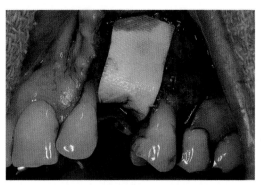

Fig. 17. Covering the bone graft site and improving incorporation of the particulate graft around the block using a collagen membrane.

The symphysis donor site offers the greatest volume of intraoral bone.[32,33] The ease of surgical access is another advantage of this region. Large blocks of bone can be harvested as well as significant quantities of particulate graft. However, the symphysis is associated with a greater incidence of postoperative complications.[32–36] These complications include neurosensory changes (lip, chin, anterior teeth), pulpal injury, concern for altered facial contour, and significant postoperative pain.[37,38]

The posterior mandible is an excellent donor site, and this area offers several advantages over the symphysis.[33,36,39] A cortical block graft approximately 4 mm in width may be harvested from the buccal aspect of the ramus region. The rectangular graft may extend up to 40 mm in length and more than 10 mm in height. This morphology is well suited for width augmentation of the narrow maxillary ridge. Both sides of the mandible may be used when significant veneer grafting is needed. The posterior mandible is also an excellent area for harvesting particulate bone with a scraper device.[40] The particulate bone can be used for sinus bone grafting and/or placed around the periphery of the bone block. The mandibular ramus has less morbidity than the symphysis and has become the preferred donor site of many clinicians.[33,35,36,40] Although there is a low risk of inferior alveolar nerve injury, this complication can be avoided by knowledge of mandibular canal anatomy and a strict adherence to the recommended osteotomies.[33,41] Compared with chin graft surgery,

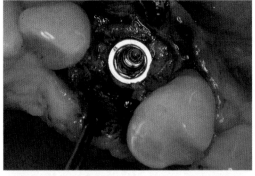

Fig. 18. Insertion of the implant after 4 months of graft healing. Favorable bone quality requires only a 2-month healing period.

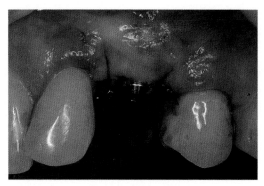

Fig. 19. Uncovering the implant after 2-month healing.

ramus grafting in patients seems to result in fewer difficulties with managing postoperative pain and also lesser concern with bone removal from this area.[33,36]

When treating large defects and advanced maxillary atrophy, larger bone grafts may be harvested from the iliac crest. Corticocancellous block bone grafts from the ilium are especially useful for reconstructing the atrophic anterior maxilla. Severe horizontal and vertical deficiencies can be managed with this approach. When thicker pieces of bone are needed for significant vertical bone augmentation, a tricortical bone graft may be harvested using the entire width of the iliac crest.[4] The use of a pain pump with a long-acting local anesthetic (bupivacaine) has dramatically reduced the level of postoperative pain from the hip area.[42] Although the proximal tibia is an attractive donor site for harvest in an office setting, the bone is mostly cancellous; so, titanium mesh or membrane techniques are needed for graft stabilization and protection.

BONE GRAFT INCORPORATION

Bone graft resorption is a necessary biologic aspect of graft healing and incorporation to the osseous recipient site. Cortical bone grafts undergo creeping substitution with replacement by new bone over time.[43] Although the embryologic origin of the bone graft was suggested as a predictor of resorption, more recent studies emphasize the importance of the osseous microarchitecture.[43–46] Denser cortical bone grafts resorb less than more porous cancellous bone grafts.[46] Cortical bone grafts from

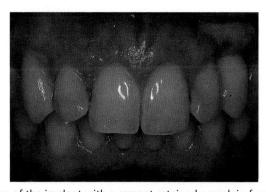

Fig. 20. Restoration of the implant with a cement-retained porcelain fused to metal crown.

the mandible exhibit minimal resorption and maintain their dense quality, making them ideal for onlay augmentation before implant placement. The volume loss of cortical bone grafts used for onlay augmentation has been measured as less than 25%.[38,47] Corticocancellous bone grafts from the ilium are associated with greater resorption because of the thinner outer cortex and more porous cancellous component.[48,49] Although some studies have reported higher rates of graft resorption, they still conclude that onlay bone grafting is a predictable technique for implant placement.[38,48,50,51] It is prudent to slightly overbuild the reconstructed ridge in anticipation of some volume loss on healing.

The use of a barrier membrane has been suggested as a strategy to reduce resorption of block bone grafts. Although some studies have found that membranes have a positive influence on graft healing, others dispute the benefit of this practice.[52] Cortical bone grafts exhibit minimal resorption and do not typically require membrane protection.[32,38,46,47,53] Although the routine use of membranes over onlay bone grafts is questionable, a barrier membrane may improve the incorporation of the peripheral particulate graft around the block.[54]

It is imperative that the onlay bone graft remains immobilized during healing. In the partially edentulous patient, a fixed provisional prosthesis, such as a temporary bridge or bonded prosthesis, is preferred for tooth replacement over the grafted site. Transitional implants have been used successfully to support fixed interim prostheses for patients less tolerant of complete or partial dentures.[55] The transitional implants should be placed in native bones and not within the bone graft. A removable Essix retainer is another excellent option for cosmetic tooth replacement during graft healing because it does not place any pressure on the site. The use of a soft tissue–borne removable prosthesis is discouraged for the first few weeks until the incision has healed. Removable prostheses should then be adjusted to minimize any contact with the grafted site. A metal base removable partial denture, with rest seats on the abutment teeth, is preferred over an acrylic soft tissue–borne prosthesis because there is less potential for loading of the graft under function. The major connector of the partial denture should be designed, so there is no metal framework over the graft site. For patients wearing a complete denture, the flange should be removed over the graft area. The internal surface of the prosthesis should also be generously relieved over the graft site. The denture may be relined with tissue conditioner after suture removal. Patients are instructed to use their removable prosthesis for cosmetic appearance and minimize function. Patients wearing removable prostheses over larger bone grafts should maintain a softer diet for at least 2 months after surgery. After this period, the onlay graft has formed a union to the host bone and relies less on the fixation screws for immobility.

Smoking has been associated with a high rate of wound dehiscence and graft failure.[56] Unless a patient commits to not smoke during the early postoperative course, onlay bone grafting is discouraged. A smoking cessation protocol is followed, including the use of prescription medications, such as bupropion, and the nicotine patch. Patients are instructed to quit smoking 1 week before surgery and told not to smoke at least until the incision is completely closed (2 weeks).[4]

IMPLANT PLACEMENT

Reconstruction of the atrophic jaws for implant placement is usually staged with implant placement after graft healing. Enough time should elapse for graft incorporation, but implants should be inserted early enough to stimulate and maintain the regenerated bone.[48] Autogenous block grafts should heal for approximately 4 months before implant placement.[32,57] The placement of implants into healed bone grafts is similar to their use in sites that have not been grafted. However, the implant site is often at the junction between the block and host bone. The surgeon should be careful not to displace the block from the ridge during the implant osteotomy and placement. Fixation screws are usually removed before implant insertion but may be left in place if they are remote. Elevation of large flaps for screw removal is discouraged because this disrupts the vascular supply to the healed graft. A small mucosal incision over the screw head allows for easy retrieval.

The integration period of implants placed into healed bone grafts is based on the resulting bone quality. Stable implants in dense cortical bone grafts (type 1–2) may only require 2-month healing. Implants placed into softer corticocancellous grafts (type 3) may need up to 4-month healing. Early Swedish studies on implants placed in iliac bone grafts found low survival rates,[58,59] which was attributed to the use of machined implants, simultaneous graft-implant placement, and a developmental learning period. Much higher implant survival can be achieved in maxillary iliac bone grafts with staged surgery and use of microtextured implants (94.5%–100%).[49,60–64] Studies on intraoral bone grafts for localized defect repair have also found very high implant survival rates (96.9%–100%).[38,65–69] Implant loading stimulates the healed bone graft and maintains the volume. Additional graft resorption following implant placement and delayed loading has not been noted radiographically.[70–72]

REFERENCES

1. Schropp L, Wenzel A, Kostopoulos L, et al. Bone healing and soft tissue contour changes following single-tooth extraction: a clinical and radiographic 12-month prospective study. Int J Periodontics Restorative Dent 2003;23:313–23.
2. Tallgren A. The continuing reduction of the residual alveolar ridges in complete denture wearers: a mixed-longitudinal study covering 25 years. J Prosthet Dent 2003;89:427–35.
3. Lekholm U, Zarb GA. Patient selection and preparation. In: Branemark P-I, Zarb GA, Albrektsson T, editors. Tissue-integrated prostheses: osseointegration in clinical dentistry. Chicago: Quintessence Publishing Co; 1985. p. 199–209.
4. Misch CM. Autogenous bone grafting for dental implants. In: Fonseca RJ, Turvery TA, Marciani RD, editors. 2nd edition, Oral and maxillofacial surgery, vol. 1. Philadelphia: W.B. Saunders Co; 2008. p. 344–70. Chapter 24.
5. Aghaloo TL, Moy PK. Which hard tissue augmentation techniques are the most successful in furnishing bony support for implant placement? Int J Oral Maxillofac Implants 2007;22(Suppl):49–70.
6. Katsoulis J, Pazera P, Mericske-Stern R. Prosthetically driven, computer-guided implant planning for the edentulous maxilla: a model study. Clin Implant Dent Relat Res 2009;11:238–45.
7. Misch CM. Use of a surgical template for autologous bone grafting of alveolar defects. J Prosthodont 1999;8(1):47–52.
8. Mecall RA, Rosenfeld AL. Influence of residual ridge resorption patterns on fixture placement and tooth position, part III: presurgical assessment of ridge augmentation requirements. Int J Periodontics Restorative Dent 1996;16:322–37.
9. Misch CE. Stress factors: influence on treatment planning. In: Misch CE, editor. Dental implant prosthetics. St Louis (MO): Mosby Inc; 2005. p. 71–90.
10. Misch CE. Maxillary sinus augmentation for endosteal implants: organized alternative treatment plans. Int J Oral Implantol 1987;4:49–58.

11. Bedrossian E, Sullivan RM, Fortin Y, et al. Fixed-prosthetic implant restoration of the edentulous maxilla: a systematic pretreatment evaluation method. J Oral Maxillofac Surg 2008;66:112–22.
12. Lindquist JW, Rockler B, Carlsson GE. Bone resorption around fixtures in edentulous patients treated with mandibular fixed tissue integrated prostheses. J Prosthet Dent 1988;59:59–63.
13. Shackleton JL, Carr L, Slabbert JC. Survival of fixed implant-supported prostheses related to cantilever lengths. J Prosthet Dent 1994;71:23–6.
14. Wyatt CC, Zarb GA. Bone level changes proximal to oral implants supporting fixed partial prostheses. Clin Oral Implants Res 2002;13:62–8.
15. Stafford GL. Survival rates of short-span implant-supported cantilever fixed dental prostheses. Evid Based Dent 2010;11:50–1.
16. Naert I, Quirynen M, Van Steenberghe D, et al. A study of 589 consecutive implants supporting complete fixed prostheses. Part II: prosthetic aspects. J Prosthet Dent 1992;68:949–56.
17. Ekfeldt A, Christiansson U, Eriksson T, et al. A retrospective analysis of factors associated with multiple implant failures in maxillae. Clin Oral Implants Res 2001;12:462–7.
18. Van der Zaag J, Lobbezoo F, Van der Avoort PG, et al. Effects of pergolide on severe sleep bruxism in a patient experiencing oral implant failure. J Oral Rehabil 2007;34:317–22.
19. Hutton EJ, Heath MR, Chai JY, et al. Factors related to success and failure rates at 3-year follow-up in a multicenter study of overdentures supported by Brånemark implants. Int J Oral Maxillofac Implants 1995;10:33–42.
20. Andreiotelli M, Att W, Strub JR. Prosthodontic complications with implant overdentures: a systematic literature review. Int J Prosthodont 2010;23:195–203.
21. Cavallaro JS, Tarnow DP. Unsplinted implants retaining maxillary overdentures with partial palatal coverage: report of 5 consecutive cases. Int J Oral Maxillofac Implants 2007;22:808–14.
22. Chan MF, Närhi TO, de Baat C, et al. Treatment of the atrophic edentulous maxilla with implant-supported overdentures: a review of the literature. Int J Prosthodont 1998;11:7–15.
23. Johns RB, Jemt T, Heath MR, et al. A multicenter study of overdentures supported by Brånemark implants. Int J Oral Maxillofac Implants 1992;7:513–22.
24. Jemt T, Book K, Lindén B, et al. Failures and complications in 92 consecutively inserted overdentures supported by Brånemark implants in severely resorbed edentulous maxillae: a study from prosthetic treatment to first annual check-up. Int J Oral Maxillofac Implants 1992;7:162–7.
25. Sanna A, Nuytens P, Naert I, et al. Successful outcome of splinted implants supporting a 'planned' maxillary overdenture: a retrospective evaluation and comparison with fixed full dental prostheses. Clin Oral Implants Res 2009;20:406–13.
26. Hooghe M, Naert I. Implant supported overdentures—the Leuven experience. J Dent 1997;25:S25–32.
27. Krennmair G, Krainhöfner M, Piehslinger E. Implant-supported maxillary overdentures retained with milled bars: maxillary anterior versus maxillary posterior concept—a retrospective study. Int J Oral Maxillofac Implants 2008;23:343–52.
28. Adell R, Lekholm U, Branemark P-I. Surgical procedures. In: Branemark P-I, Zarb GA, Albrektsson T, editors. Tissue-integrated prostheses: osseointegration in clinical dentistry. Chicago: Quintessence Publishing Co; 1985. p. 211–32.

29. Brånemark PI, Svensson B, van Steenberghe D. Ten-year survival rates of fixed prostheses on four or six implants ad modum Brånemark in full edentulism. Clin Oral Implants Res 1995;6:227–31.
30. Maló P, Rangert B, Nobre M. All-on-4 immediate-function concept with Brånemark System implants for completely edentulous maxillae: a 1-year retrospective clinical study. Clin Implant Dent Relat Res 2005;7(Suppl 1):S88–94.
31. Balshi TJ, Wolfinger GJ. Immediate loading of dental implants in the edentulous maxilla: case study of a unique protocol. Int J Periodontics Restorative Dent 2003; 23:37–45.
32. Misch CM, Misch CE, Resnik RR, et al. Reconstruction of maxillary alveolar defects with mandibular symphysis grafts for dental implants: a preliminary procedural report. Int J Oral Maxillofac Implants 1992;7:360–6.
33. Misch CM. Comparison of intraoral donor sites for onlay grafting prior to implant placement. Int J Oral Maxillofac Implants 1997;12:767–76.
34. Raghoebar GM, Louwerse C, Kalk WW. Morbidity of chin bone harvesting. Clin Oral Implants Res 2001;12:503–7.
35. Nkenke E, Schulze-Mosgau S, Radespiel M. Morbidity of harvesting of chin grafts: a prospective study. Clin Oral Implants Res 2001;12:495–502.
36. Hallman M, Hedin M, Sennerby L. A prospective 1 year clinical and radiographic study of implants placed after maxillary sinus floor augmentation with bovine hydroxyapatite and autogenous bone. J Oral Maxillofac Surg 2002;60:277–84.
37. Jensen J, Sindet-Pedersen S. Autogenous mandibular bone grafts and osseointegrated implants for reconstruction of severely atrophied maxilla: a preliminary report. J Oral Maxillofac Surg 1991;49:1277–87.
38. Cordaro L, Amadé DS, Cordaro M. Clinical results of alveolar ridge augmentation with mandibular block bone grafts in partially edentulous patients prior to implant placement. Clin Oral Implants Res 2002;13:103–11.
39. Misch CM. Ridge augmentation using mandibular ramus bone grafts for the placement of dental implants: presentation of a technique. Pract Periodontics Aesthet Dent 1996;8:127–35.
40. Peleg M, Garg AK, Misch CM, et al. Maxillary sinus and ridge augmentations using a surface-derived autogenous bone graft. J Oral Maxillofac Surg 2004; 62:1535–44.
41. Misch CM. Use of the mandibular ramus as a donor site for onlay bone grafting. J Oral Implantol 2000;26:42–9.
42. Hoard MA, Bill TJ, Campbell RL. Reduction in morbidity after iliac crest bone harvesting: the concept of preemptive analgesia. J Craniofac Surg 1998;9:448–51.
43. Manson PN. Facial bone healing and bone grafts. A review of clinical physiology. Clin Plast Surg 1994;21:331–48.
44. Smith JD, Abramson M. Membranous vs endochondral autografts. Arch Otolaryngol 1974;99:203–9.
45. Zins JE, Whitaker LA. Membranous vs endochondral autografts: implications for craniofacial reconstruction. Plast Reconstr Surg 1983;72:778–85.
46. Ozaki W, Buchman SR. Volume maintenance of onlay bone grafts in the craniofacial skeleton: micro-architecture versus embryologic origin. Plast Reconstr Surg 1998;102:291–9.
47. Proussaefs P, Lozada J, Kleinman A. The use of ramus autogenous block grafts for vertical alveolar ridge augmentation and implant placement: a pilot study. Int J Oral Maxillofac Implants 2002;17:238–48.
48. Nystrom E, Ahlqvist J, Kahnberg KE, et al. Autogenous onlay bone grafts fixed with screw implants for the treatment of severely resorbed maxillae. Radiographic

evaluation of preoperative bone dimensions, postoperative bone loss, and changes in soft-tissue profile. Int J Oral Maxillofac Surg 1996;25:351–9.

49. Reinert S, Konig S, Bremerich A, et al. Stability of bone grafting and placement of implants in the severely atrophic maxilla. Br J Oral Maxillofac Surg 2003;41: 249–55.

50. Widmark G, Andersson B, Ivanoff CJ. Mandibular bone graft in the anterior maxilla for single-tooth implants. Int J Oral Maxillofac Surg 1997;26:106–9.

51. Sbordone L, Toti P, Menchini-Fabris GB, et al. Volume changes of autogenous bone grafts after alveolar ridge augmentation of atrophic maxillae and mandibles. Int J Oral Maxillofac Surg 2009;38:1059–65.

52. Gielkens PF, Bos RR, Raghoebar GM, et al. Is there evidence that barrier membranes prevent bone resorption in autologous bone grafts during the healing period? A systematic review. Int J Oral Maxillofac Implants 2007;22:390–8.

53. Dongieux JW, Block MS, Morris G, et al. The effect of different membranes on on-lay bone graft success in the dog mandible. Oral Surg Oral Med Oral Pathol Oral Radiol Endod 1998;86:145–51.

54. Buser D, Dula K, Hirt HP, et al. Lateral ridge augmentation using autografts and barrier membranes: a clinical study with 40 partially edentulous patients. J Oral Maxillofac Surg 1996;54:420–32.

55. Krennmair G, Krainhofner M, Weinlander M. Provisional implants for immediate restoration of partially edentulous jaws: a clinical study. Int J Oral Maxillofac Implants 2008;23:717–25.

56. Levin L, Schwartz-Arad D. The effect of cigarette smoking on dental implants and related surgery. Implant Dent 2005;14:357–61.

57. Matsumoto MA, Filho HN, Francishone CE. Microscopic analysis of reconstructed maxillary alveolar ridges using autogenous bone grafts from the chin and iliac crest. Int J Oral Maxillofac Implants 2002;17:507–16.

58. Breine U, Branemark PI. Reconstruction of alveolar jaw bone. An experimental and clinical study of immediate and preformed autologous bone grafts in combination with osseointegrated implants. Scand J Plast Reconstr Surg 1980;14:23–48.

59. Adell R, Lekholm U, Grondahl K, et al. Reconstruction of severely resorbed eden-tulous maxillae using osseointegrated fixtures in immediate autogenous bone grafts. Int J Oral Maxillofac Implants 1990;5:233–46.

60. Misch CE, Dietsh F. Endosteal implants and iliac crest grafts to restore severely resorbed totally edentulous maxillae—a retrospective study. J Oral Implantol 1994;20:100–10.

61. Verhoeven JW, Cune MS, Terlou M, et al. The combined use of endosteal implants and iliac crest onlay grafts in the severely atrophic mandible: a longitudinal study. Int J Oral Maxillofac Surg 1997;26:351–7.

62. Joos U, Kleinheinz J. Reconstruction of the severely resorbed (Class VI) jaws: routine of exception? J Craniomaxillofac Surg 2000;28:1–4.

63. Thor A, Wannfors K, Sennerby L, et al. Reconstruction of the severely resorbed maxilla with autogenous bone, platelet-rich plasma and implants: 1-year results of a controlled prospective 5-year study. Clin Implant Dent Relat Res 2005;7: 209–20.

64. Nelson K, Ozyuvaci H, Bilgic B, et al. Histomorphometric evaluation and clinical assessment of endosseous implants in iliac bone grafts with shortened healing periods. Int J Oral Maxillofac Implants 2006;21:392–8.

65. Raghoebar GM, Batenburg RH, Vissink A, et al. Augmentation of localized defects of the anterior maxillary ridge with autogenous bone before insertion of implants. J Oral Maxillofac Surg 1996;54:1180–5.

66. Von Arx T, Wallkamm B, Hardt N. Localized ridge augmentation using a micro tita-
    nium mesh: a report on 27 implants followed 1 to 3 years after functional loading.
    Clin Oral Implants Res 1998;9:123–30.
67. Sethi A, Kaus T. Ridge augmentation using mandibular block bone grafts: prelim-
    inary results of an ongoing prospective study. Int J Oral Maxillofac Implants 2001;
    16:378–88.
68. Zerbo I, de Lange G, Joldersma M, et al. Fate of monocortical bone blocks
    grafted in the human maxilla: a histological and histomorphometric study. Clin
    Oral Implants Res 2003;14:759–66.
69. Levin L, Nitzan D, Schwartz-Arad D. Success of dental implants placed in intrao-
    ral block bone grafts. J Periodontol 2007;78:18–21.
70. Buser D, Ingimarsson S, Dula K. Long term stability of osseointegrated implants
    in augmented bone: a 5-year prospective study in partially edentulous patients.
    Int J Periodontics Restorative Dent 2002;22:108–17.
71. Sbordone L, Toti P, Menchini-Fabris G, et al. Implant survival in maxillary and
    mandibular osseous onlay grafts and native bone: a 3-year clinical and comput-
    erized tomographic follow-up. Int J Oral Maxillofac Implants 2009;24:695–703.
72. Nyström E, Nilson H, Gunne J, et al. A 9–14 year follow-up of onlay bone grafting
    in the atrophic maxilla. Int J Oral Maxillofac Surg 2009;38:111–6.

Guided Surgery for Implant Therapy

Gary Orentlicher, DMD[a,b,*], Marcus Abboud, DMD[c]

KEYWORDS

- Guided surgery • Dental implant • Flapless surgery
- CT/CBCT scans

With the recent introduction of new three-dimensional (3D) diagnostic and treatment planning technologies in implant dentistry, a team approach to the planning and place-ment of dental implants, according to a restoratively driven treatment plan, has become the norm in quality patient care. The team can now start with the end result, the planned tooth, and then place an implant into the correct position according to the restorative plan. The accurate and predictable placement of implants according to a computer-generated virtual treatment plan is now a reality, taking the virtual plan from the computer to the patient clinically. Recent advances in 3D imaging in dentistry, in combination with the introduction of third-party proprietary implant planning soft-ware and associated surgical instrumentation, have revolutionized dental implant diagnosis and treatment and created an interdisciplinary environment in which communication leads to better patient care and outcomes.

HISTORICAL OVERVIEW

Since the introduction of the first dental radiographs, dentists have become comfort-able with evaluating and diagnosing patients using two-dimensional (2D) images (ie, periapical, bitewing, panoramic, and cephalometric radiographs, and so forth). The obvious limitations of these technologies in evaluating 3D problems required clinician acceptance because few options were available. Because of their hospital-based training, oral and maxillofacial surgeons have long used computed tomography (CT) scans for the 3D evaluation of facial trauma and pathologic lesions. These CT evalu-ations typically were viewed in 2D as axial or reformatted frontal or coronal slices

This article was previously published in the May 2011 issue of *Oral and Maxillofacial Surgery Clinics of North America*.

[a] Private Practice, New York Oral, Maxillofacial, and Implant Surgery, 495 Central Park Avenue, Suite 201, Scarsdale, NY 10583, USA

[b] Oral and Maxillofacial Surgery, White Plains Hospital, White Plains, NY, USA

[c] Department of Prosthodontics and Digital Technology, Stony Brook University School of Dental Medicine, 160 Rockland Hall, Stony Brook, NY 11794-8700 , USA

* Corresponding author. Private Practice, New York Oral, Maxillofacial, and Implant Surgery, 495 Central Park Avenue, Suite 201, NY 10583.

E-mail address: drgaryo@yahoo.com

Dent Clin N Am 55 (2011) 715–744

doi:10.1016/j.cden.2011.07.008

0011-8532/11/$ – see front matter © 2011 Elsevier Inc. All rights reserved.

dental.theclinics.com

through the area of interest of a patient's anatomy, printed on plain films, or viewed as such on a computer screen. The remainder of the dental community had little, if any, exposure to 3D image evaluation.

The first medical-grade helical CT scanners were all single-slice, slower machines that were based in hospitals or private radiology facilities. Typical medical multislice CT scanners of today are capable of performing a scan of the upper and/or lower jaw in a few seconds, but the size and cost of the machines, the radiation exposure, the lack of familiarity and training amongst dentists, and the perceived cost/benefit ratio in patient care made them inappropriate for a dental office setting. With the development and introduction of the New Tom 9000 (Quantitative Radiology, Verona, Italy) in 1998, cone beam volumetric tomography (CBVT/cone beam computed tomography [CBCT]) was introduced to the dental community.[1] Although the first machines were larger than those available today, the advantages were that they produced good 3D images at lower radiation doses,[2–4] and the footprint of the machines were small enough to fit into a dental office. The disadvantages were that, although the radiation was less than medical-grade CT, it was more than conventional dental radiographs and, because of the reduced radiation, the images produced had less definition than medical CT. Since the first CBCT was introduced, machines with multiple different features have been developed and introduced by various manufacturers. The gold standard for accurate 3D diagnosis continues to be medical-grade CT.[5,6] The recent introduction of adaptive statistical iterative reconstruction (ASIR) software has been reported to allow up to a 50% radiation dose reduction in medical CT scans, without diminishing image quality.[7–10] There are different average deviations and percentage error measurements for all CBCT scanners.[11,12]

In the late 1980s, articles began to appear in the literature discussing the use of DentaScans to evaluate the bone of the maxilla and mandible in preparation for placement of dental implants.[13–16] Columbia Scientific (CSI) introduced the 3D Dental software in 1988. This software converted CT axial slices into reformatted cross-sectional images of the alveolar ridges for diagnosis and evaluation. In 1991, a combination software was introduced, ImageMaster-101, which allowed the additional feature of placing graphic dental implants on the cross-sectional images. The first version of Sim/Plant was introduced by CSI in 1993, allowing the placement of virtual implants of exact dimensions, on CT images, in cross-sectional, axial, and panoramic views. In 1999, Simplant 6.0 was introduced, adding the creation of 3D reformatted image surface rendering to the software.[17] Materialise (Leuven, Belgium) purchased CSI in 2001, introducing the technology for drilling osteotomies to exact depth and direction through a surgical guide in 2002. NobelBiocare (Zurich, Switzerland) introduced the NobelProcera/NobelGuide technology in 2005. The NobelGuide technology was introduced as a complete implant planning and placement system, for both straight-walled and tapered NobelBiocare implants. Appropriate instrumentation was developed to create osteotomies of accurate depth and direction, as well as the ability to place implants flapless, to accurate depth, through a guide. The system was designed for conventional postimplant insertion treatment (cover screws or healing abutments), immediate loading of implants, and the fabrication of partial or full arch restorations before implant placement. A completely redesigned upgrade of the NobelGuide software, NobelClinician, has been introduced in 2011. Software from other manufacturers, such as EasyGuide (Keystone Dental, Burlington, MA, USA), Straumann coDiagnostiX (Straumann, Basel, Switzerland), VIP Software (BioHorizons, Birmingham, AL, USA), Implant Master (IDent, Foster City, CA, USA), and others, are now available as well. Other implant manufacturers have developed instrument trays for the guided placement of their implants using the Simplant software for implant planning (ie, Facilitate, AstraTech Dental, Molndal, Sweden; Navigator, Biomet 3i, Palm Beach Gardens, FL, USA; ExpertEase, Dentsply Friadent, Mannheim, Germany.)

GENERAL TECHNOLOGY CONCEPTS

CT/CBCT scanners allow the dentist and surgeon to visualize a patient's anatomy in 3 dimensions. Visualization of the height and width of available bone for implant placement, soft tissue thicknesses, proximity and root anatomy of adjacent teeth, the exact location of the maxillary sinuses, and other pertinent vital structures such as the mandibular canal, mental foramen, and incisive canal are possible.[18–20] Once images are imported into proprietary software programs (eg, Simplant, NobelClinician) the clinician can then virtually treatment plan the placement of implants for an individual patient's anatomy and case plan. The type and size of the planned implant, its position within the bone, its relationship to the planned restoration and adjacent teeth and/or implants, and its proximity to vital structures can be determined before performing surgery.[18–22] Computer-generated surgical drilling guides can then be fabricated from the virtual treatment plan. These surgical guides are used by the doctor to place the planned implants in the patient's mouth in the same positions as in the virtual treatment plan, allowing more accurate and predictable implant placement[23–27] and reduced patient morbidity.[28–31]

All of the current systems have similar restorative and surgical protocols. Upper and lower arch impressions are made and a bite registration is obtained. Models are poured and mounted on an articulator. Guided surgery requires reverse planning. The prosthodontist or restorative dentist first creates an ideal restorative treatment plan, determining the planned tooth position by creating a diagnostic wax-up that indicates the exact anatomy and position of the teeth to be replaced. An acrylic prosthesis is then fabricated that reproduces the planned restorations in the acrylic appliance. Depending on the system to be used, this scan prosthesis can be a partial or full denture (**Figs. 1–3**). Most systems, other than NobelGuide, require that the planned restorations contain a 20% to 30% barium sulfate mixture in the acrylic to allow for radiopacity of the planned restorations in the CT/CBCT images. NobelGuide uses a double-scan technique with a hard acrylic scan prosthesis and gutta percha marker reference points, with no barium sulfate. The CT/CBCT scan is then taken with the patient wearing the scan prosthesis according to the individual system protocols.

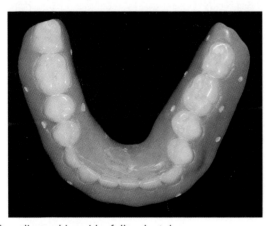

Fig. 1. NobelGuide radiographic guide, fully edentulous.

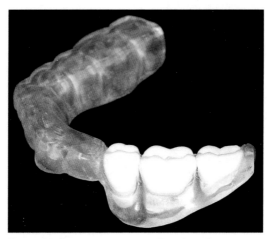

Fig. 2. Simplant radiographic barium stent, partially edentulous.

The CT scan (Digital Imaging and Communication in Medicine [DICOM]) images are then imported into the various proprietary software programs (eg, Simplant, Nobel-Guide, EasyGuide). The software programs are then used to virtually place implants into their ideal positions related to the planned restoration and the underlying bony

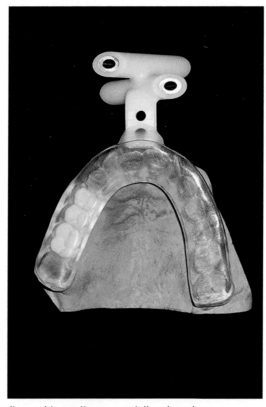

Fig. 3. EZ Guide radiographic appliance, partially edentulous.

anatomy (**Figs. 4–6**). The digital treatment plan is then uploaded to the manufacturer for fabrication of a surgical guide (**Figs. 7–9**). The surgical guide is used, with implant-specific drilling instrumentation, to precisely place the implants in the same positions, depths, and angulations as was planned virtually.

Many CT-guided implant planning technologies require radiopaque fiducial reference markers to be placed in the scan prosthesis that the patient wears during the CT/CBCT scan. These reference markers are then used by the software to virtually position the scanning appliance and, with it, the parameters of the planned restoration(s) as related to the patient's jaw. Some CBCT scanners have difficulty in accurately assessing these geometric markers. This problem has the potential to add error into a precise planning system. This error can lead to inaccurately fitting surgical guides and error in implant placement. It is advisable to make every effort to investigate and use CBCT scanners that have high levels of accuracy or medical CT scanners when using these technologies.[32]

INDICATIONS FOR USE

Because of its precision and accuracy in implant placement, an argument could be made for the use of CT-guided implant surgery in almost all cases. As with anything in medicine, a cost/time/benefit determination must be made by the clinician based on the circumstances of an individual case. The increased patient and treatment planning time, the additional expense, and the additional patient radiation exposure may outweigh the clinical benefits in certain cases. We have found that these technologies are most beneficial to the patient and the doctor in the following clinical situations:

Three or more implants in a row
Proximity to vital anatomic structures
Problems related to the proximity of adjacent teeth
Questionable bone volume
Implant position that is critical to the planned restoration
Flapless implant placement
Multiple unit or full arch immediate restorations, with or without extractions and immediate placement

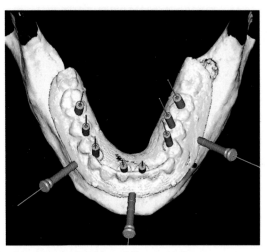

Fig. 4. NobelGuide virtual treatment plan, fully edentulous.

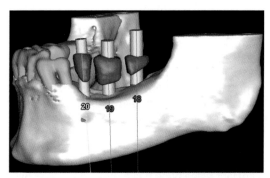

Fig. 5. Simplant virtual treatment plan, partially edentulous.

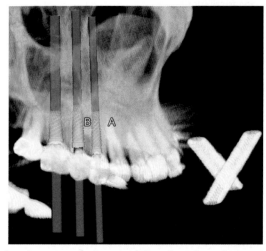

Fig. 6. EZ Guide virtual treatment plan, partially edentulous. "A" and "B" on image are associated with software measurement tool.

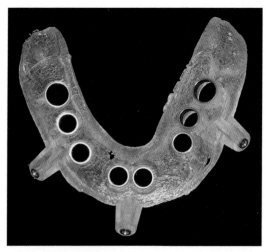

Fig. 7. NobelBiocare NobelGuide fabricated from treatment plan, **Figs. 1** and **4**.

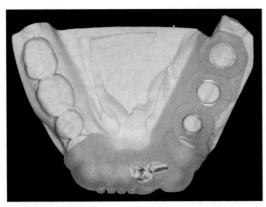

Fig. 8. Simplant SurgiGuide fabricated from treatment plan, Figs. 2 and 5.

Significant alteration of the soft tissue or bony anatomy by prior surgery or trauma
Patients with physical, medical, and psychiatric comorbidities.

Conventional surgical stents to aid in implant positioning have been used in implant
dentistry for many years. Guides of these types can be simple (ie, vacuform shells with
the buccal or palatal/lingual facings of the planned restorations) or more complex (ie,
stents with 2-mm drill holes or metal tubes). The problem is that there is no correlation
in these appliances between the planned restoration and the underlying bony
anatomy. With the use of computer-guided implant surgical guides, this anatomic relationship can be predictably established and considered before surgery.

The fabrication of a surgical guide, used in implant treatment, is determined by the
patient's anatomy and local references, such as the numbers and locations of teeth in
the arch to be treated or in the opposing arch. With increasing length of the edentulous
area, fewer anatomic references are present for the predictable accurate placement of
implants. In a fully edentulous case, other than the soft tissue ridge and palate, all local
references are lost. Bone and soft tissue loss from periodontal disease and atrophy,
long-term denture wear, and sinus pneumatization can make it difficult to predictably
use a traditional surgical guide.

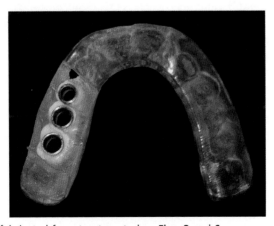

Fig. 9. EZ Guide fabricated from treatment plan, Figs. 3 and 6.

In cases in which 3 or more implants in a row are planned, concepts of implant spacing and angulations, implant parallelism in all dimensions, proximity of implants to anatomic structures, and relationships between implant positions and the planned restorations are significant considerations for the clinician. CT/CBCT-guided surgery allows for the ideal placement of multiple dental implants according to the planned restoration, the relationships of implants to surrounding anatomy, and principles of ideal implant positioning and spacing (**Figs. 10–13**).

Differences in radiograph machines and radiographic techniques commonly lead to distortion of anatomic structures on conventional 2D images, such as elongation, shortening, stretching, and contraction. Accurate 3D evaluations and measurements of the relationship between a planned implant and the position of the mental nerve, inferior alveolar nerve (**Figs. 14** and **15**), nasopalatine/incisive nerve (**Fig. 16**), maxillary sinuses, and nasal floor (**Fig. 17**) are best visualized, evaluated, and measured by using CT-generated images. In cases in which there are questions of nerve or sinus proximity related to the patient's available bone, implants are most accurately placed using computer-generated surgical guides. These technologies minimize potential patient morbidities.

All proprietary implant planning softwares have the functionality to isolate the roots of teeth in the edentulous areas to aid in the accurate placement of implants between and adjacent to tooth roots in the planned sites. Some softwares use virtual dots or lines to outline tooth roots (**Fig. 18**), whereas others have the ability to alter the software's sensitivity to Hounsfield units or isovalues to virtually remove bone from around tooth roots (called segmentation) (**Fig. 19**). These technologies are most beneficial when tooth roots are in extremely divergent or convergent relationships or when implants must be placed in tight spaces because of close root proximities.

Surgical dilemmas that require implant placement in only 1 location, and/or at only 1 implant depth, are common. Difficult clinical scenarios frequently require the placement of implants into tight spaces with minimal bony leeway either mesial-distally, buccal-lingually, or both (see **Fig. 16**; **Fig. 20**). Adjacent tooth root proximity can make implant placement feel to the clinician like threading a needle. This is a common problem with congenitally missing teeth. Scenarios of limited bone volume often leave situations in which the patient's anatomy dictates where the implant can be placed. Essentially, there is only 1 location in which an implant can be placed.

Some of the most complex restorative and surgical cases treated in implant dentistry involve single and multiple implants in the esthetic zone. Thicknesses of crestal and buccal soft tissues and buccal and palatal cortical plates, buccal-lingual

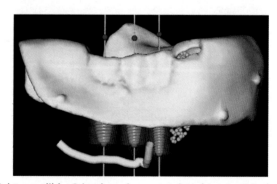

Fig. 10. Lower right mandible, 3 implants in a row, virtual treatment plan.

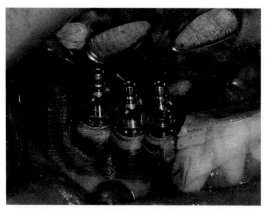

Fig. 11. Three implants in a row, NobelGuide in place. Note implant mounts with attached implants placed to depth.

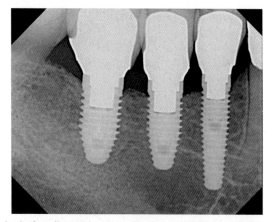

Fig. 12. Final periapical radiograph. Note implant parallelism, different diameters and lengths, and spacing corresponding to the implant site and the planned restorations.

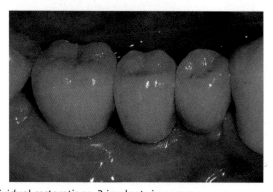

Fig. 13. Final individual restorations, 3 implants in a row.

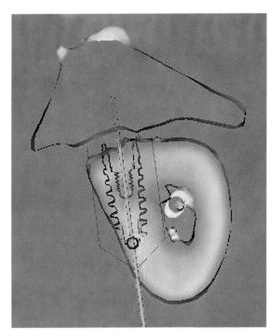

Fig. 14. Severe atrophy posterior mandible, implant placement planned lingual to the inferior alveolar nerve.

ridge dimensions, proximity to adjacent teeth, implant-to-root relationships, gingival and papilla support and contours, gingival exposure, smile lines, and implant angulations and emergence are just a few of the many complex considerations. In addition, knowledge of the appropriate implant position based on the type of restoration

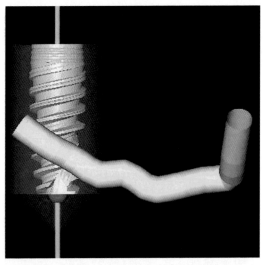

Fig. 15. 3D reformation of **Fig. 14.** Note appearance of proximity between implant and inferior alveolar nerve in lateral view.

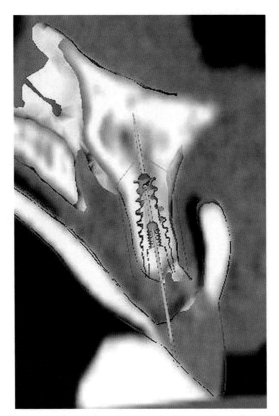

Fig. 16. Implant placement planned in close proximity to enlarged nasopalatine canal.

planned (ie, cement or screw retained) is an important prosthetic-based consideration. Very small variations in implant positions can lead to difficult restorative dilemmas in these cases. Proper implant position can be critical to the esthetic and functional success of the planned restoration. CT/CBCT-guided implant planning and placement allows for the evaluation and visualization of the ideal restoration for

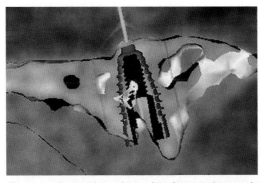

Fig. 17. Severe maxillary atrophy. Implant planned in the anterior nasal spine, in close proximity to the nasal floor.

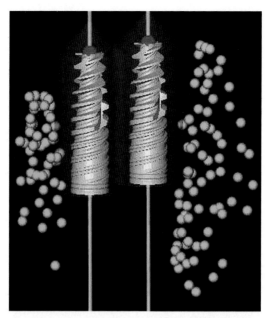

Fig. 18. Outlining of tooth roots with virtual treatment planning.

a site based on the surrounding bony and soft tissue anatomy, then the virtual placement of implants based on the planned restoration related to the underlying bone. Surgical guides then position the implants accurately and predictably into the optimal position for the planned restoration (**Figs. 21–24**).

Implant technologies and surface characteristics in use today have dramatically reduced the time required from implant placement to loading. Immediate placement and immediate loading of implants is now commonly performed. In some cases, teeth can be extracted, implants can be placed immediately, and temporary crowns can be placed at the time of implant insertion. Concepts of cross-arch stabilization and loading of multiple implants have changed the way treatment is planned. Depending on the clinical circumstances and the experience and comfort level of the dental

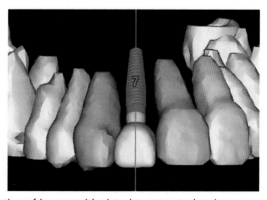

Fig. 19. Segmentation of images with virtual treatment planning.

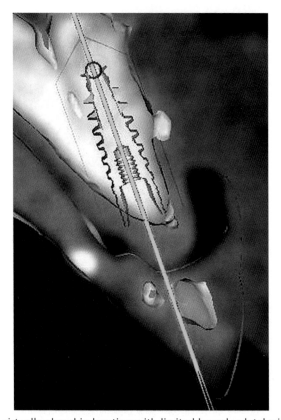

Fig. 20. Implant virtually placed in location with limited buccal-palatal width.

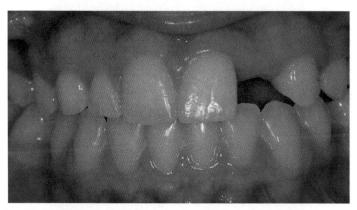

Fig. 21. Figs. 21–24: 17 year old female, over-retained maxillary right primary canine and lateral incisors and congenitally missing right canine and bilateral lateral incisors and second premolars. Preoperative grafting procedures were necessary to prepare each site for dental implants. A 17-year-old girl before surgery.

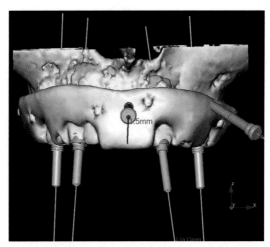

Fig. 22. Virtual treatment plan.

team, these technologies can be used to place single units, multiple units, or full arches of implants. Implants can be placed as a 2-stage, a single-stage with healing abutments, or as an immediate-placement/immediate-load case. Implants can be placed accurately with a tissue incision or flapless. Patients experience less surgical trauma, pain, and swelling. Recovery time is reduced and the return to their normal lives is expedited.[22–29]

Taking CT-guided technology to the next step involves accurate fabrication of a provisional restoration before implant insertion, with immediate insertion at the time of surgery. After the virtual treatment plan is created by the clinician (**Figs. 26** and **33**), computer-generated stereolithographic surgical guides are fabricated by

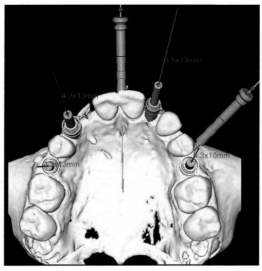

Fig. 23. Virtual treatment plan, occlusal view. Note implant planned in the right canine site for 2 unit cantilever bridge anteriorly.

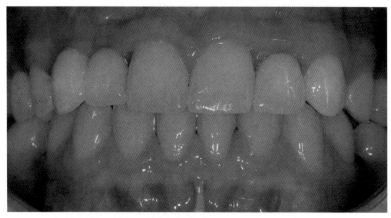

Fig. 24. The 17-year-old female from **Fig. 21**, final restorations.

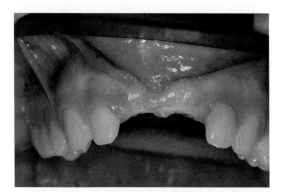

Fig. 25. Figs. 25–31: A 20-year-old man bilateral maxillary central incisors avulsed traumatically. Treatment using AstraTech Dental Facilitate technology. A 20-year-old man before surgery.

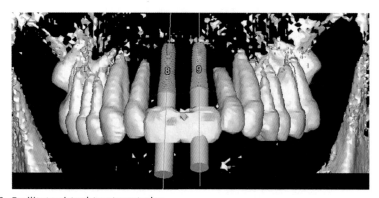

Fig. 26. Facilitate virtual treatment plan.

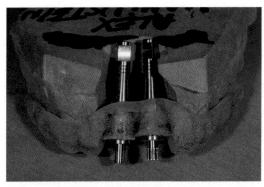

Fig. 27. Presurgical laboratory placement of implant analogs into the Facilitate surgical guide, before pouring stone into the guide for fabrication of a master model.

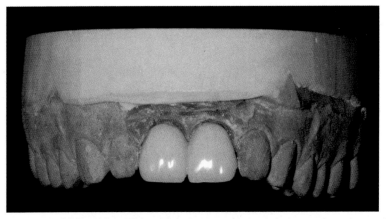

Fig. 28. Presurgical fabrication of provisional restorations on the poured master model.

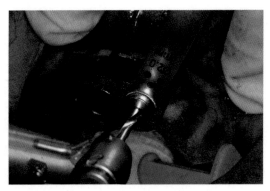

Fig. 29. Guided osteotomy preparation using the Facilitate instrumentation.

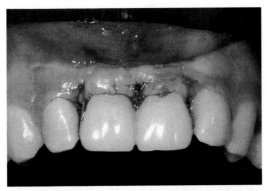

Fig. 30. Implants inserted, temporary restoration placed at the time of surgery.

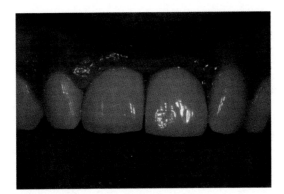

Fig. 31. Final restorations in place, 5 months later.

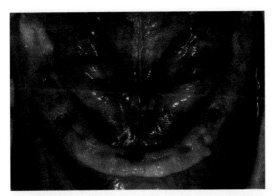

Fig. 32. Figs. 32–40: A 60-year-old man, fully edentulous mandible. The patient desired immediate fixed restorations and, ultimately, as many fixed individual crowns as possible. Preoperative mandibular ridge. Note areas where temporary implants have been removed.

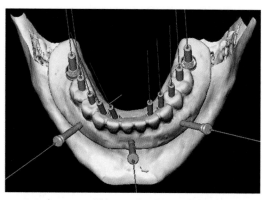

Fig. 33. Virtual treatment plan, mandible. Tenimplants planned.

the manufacturer from the virtual treatment plan (**Figs. 27** and **34**). A dental laboratory then uses the fabricated surgical guide, along with mounted patient models, to fabricate temporary, and in some cases final, restorations, before implant placement surgery (see **Figs. 27, 28, 35, 36**). The surgical guide can then be used to place implants flapless, only removing a core of tissue in the planned implant sites. Typically, once the surgical guide is accurately secured, implants can be placed through the surgical guide without removing it until all implants are inserted to proper depth and direction (**Figs. 29** and **38**). Abutments can then be immediately placed on the implants, and temporary or, in some cases, final restorations inserted (see **Figs. 25–31** and **32–40**).

In most circumstances, placing the implants where the bone is has become an outdated concept. Current techniques allow the surgeon to perform soft tissue and bone augmentation procedures to prepare the planned implant site before placing implants. Large and small soft tissue and connective tissue grafts, as well as sinus floor grafts, block grafts, alveolar ridge splits, and alveolar distraction procedures, are a few of the procedures routinely performed to prepare the recipient jaw before placing implants.

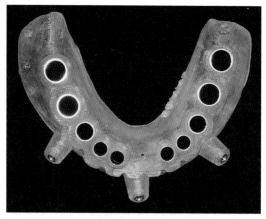

Fig. 34. NobelGuide fabricated from the virtual treatment plan.

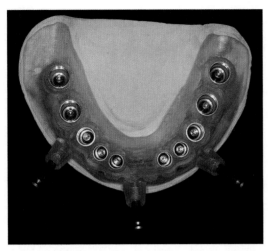

Fig. 35. Presurgical master model fabricated from the NobelGuide. Note implant analogs with temporary abutments in place.

Previous surgical procedures, including prior placement of different types of dental implants (ie, blade and subperiosteal implants), can leave patients with challenging reconstructive bony defects (**Figs. 41** and **42**). Loss of bone, teeth, and soft tissue, with resultant defects of varying sizes, can result from traumatic injuries or benign and malignant abnormalities of the jaws. Reconstructive procedures to treat these defects can leave areas of abnormal bony anatomy and scarred soft tissue. After healing, graft maturation, and settling of graft materials, resultant bone and soft tissue volumes can be unpredictable. Lateral block-onlay grafts can resorb a portion of their bone volume during healing and maturation.[33–35] CT/CBCT-guided technologies allow the surgeon to predict the volume of sinus graft material necessary to augment an area of the maxilla to a desired height of bone.[36] Newer technologies are being investigated and developed in which customized block bone grafts can be created after evaluating bony defects from CT/CBCT data.

Using these technologies allows for the visualization and evaluation of distorted anatomy without making an incision.[37] Implants can be placed accurately and

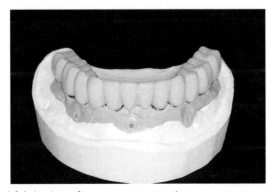

Fig. 36. Presurgical fabrication of temporary restoration.

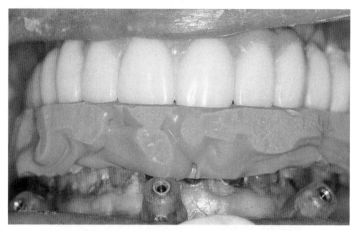

Fig. 37. Accurate surgical positioning of the NobelGuide using a surgical index (a bite registration, made on mounted models, which relates the position of the surgical guide to the opposing arch) before guide pin/screw stabilization.

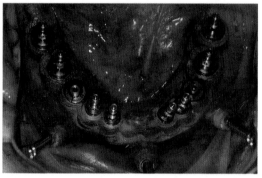

Fig. 38. Surgical guide in place with 10 implants placed to correct depth using appropriate guided instrumentation.

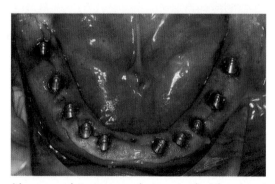

Fig. 39. Surgical guide removed, temporary abutments placed on inserted implants.

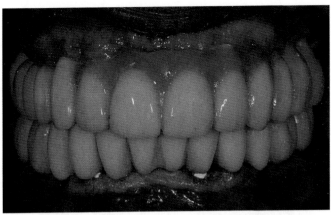

Fig. 40. Temporary full arch mandibular restoration immediately inserted at the time of surgery.

predictably with a clear knowledge of available bony anatomy, without flapping and removing periosteal blood supply (**Figs. 43–46**).

COMPROMISED PATIENTS

Pre- and postoperative radiation therapy potentially alters healing capacities in patients who have head and neck cancers. The literature advocates pre- and postoperative courses of hyperbaric oxygen therapy (HBO) to increase bone vascularity before implant placement in these patients.[38–41] Placing implants with minimal flap elevation and hard and soft tissue trauma is indicated in these patients to minimize the likelihood of the development of osteoradionecrosis.[38,42] Bleeding, swelling, and alteration of the blood supply are limited by using these technologies.[43]

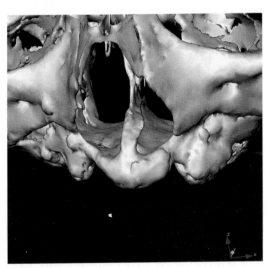

Fig. 41. A 68-year-old woman who had a prior full arch maxillary subperiosteal implant. Note severe atrophy and distorted anatomy.

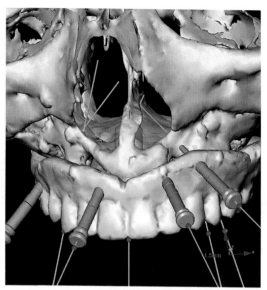

Fig. 42. Virtual treatment plan, for the case shown in **Fig. 41**, 4 implants planned for overdenture restoration.

Patients with associated medical problems, such as bleeding dyscrasias, anticoagulation issues, or significant cardiovascular disease, may require specific medication protocols that cannot be altered before surgery. Minimizing bleeding by limiting surgical trauma to the soft and hard tissues is indicated in patients with difficult

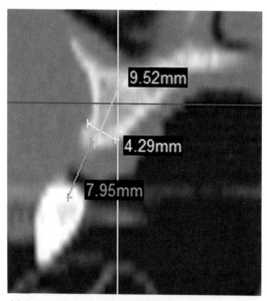

Fig. 43. A 32-year-old man, severe atrophy anterior maxilla from a sports injury. Preoperative cross-sectional image in area of right lateral incisor, Simplant. Note measurements revealing deficiencies of bone in all dimensions.

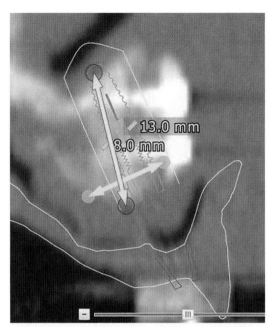

Fig. 44. Postgrafting cross-sectional image of the case shown in **Fig. 43**, area of right lateral incisor, after maxillary anterior distraction osteogenesis and lateral block grafts, NobelClinician. Note measurements of 13.0 mm (height) and 8.0 mm (width).

medical management issues. 3D implant evaluation and planning, with CT-guided implant placement, allows for flapless, minimally traumatic, accurate implant placement, an indication for use in patients with these challenging medical management problems.

Patient's historical experiences in dental offices vary greatly. Procedures that require long periods in a dental chair can prevent some patients from seeking treatment because of extreme levels of anxiety, stress, and phobias. Orthopedic and spinal disorders may limit the amount of time a patient can sit in a dental chair. Wheelchair-bound patients pose another set of logistical treatment problems. These types of patients can require extensive planning and preparation before treatment. Treatment must be performed quickly and efficiently, without compromising quality. Computer-generated implant planning allows for the preoperative visualization of most of the potential planning and anatomic issues that may be encountered during surgery, all before the patient sits in the dental chair. By using surgical guides, implants can be placed quickly and predictably, thus minimizing patient stress, pain, and time in the dental chair.

DISCUSSION

Three types of computer-generated surgical guides are currently available: tooth supported, mucosa supported, and bone supported. Tooth-supported guides are used in partially edentulous cases. The surgical guide is designed to rest on other teeth in the arch for accuracy of guide fit. Mucosal-supported guides are used primarily in fully edentulous cases and are designed to rest on the mucosa. Accurate interarch bite registrations are of utmost importance when using these guides to assure accurate

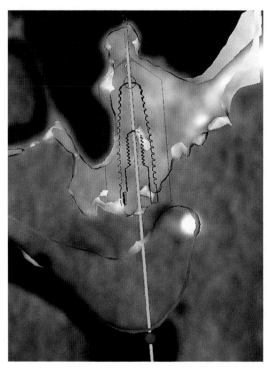

Fig. 45. Cross-sectional view, after sinus lift graft. Note bone graft placement primarily laterally, virtual implant placed.

surgical guide positioning and placement of securing screws or pins before the placement of implants (see **Fig. 37**). Bone-supported guides can be used in partially or fully edentulous cases, but are used primarily in fully edentulous cases in which significant ridge atrophy is present and good seating of a mucosa-supported guide is questionable. These guides require elevation of an extensive full-thickness flap to expose the bone in the planned implant sites and in the adjacent areas for full, stable seating of the guide over the bony ridge. At this time, only Simplant (Materialise) manufactures bone-supported surgical guides.

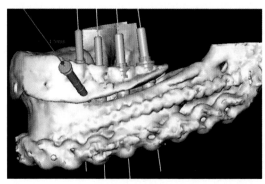

Fig. 46. 3D reconstruction of left mandible after ameloblastoma resection and iliac crest reconstruction. Virtual treatment plan, 4 implants.

Dental implant placement using CT-guided surgery with drill guides is known to enhance safety compared with using a freehand technique.[44–46] According to the NobelGuide protocol, when using the Guided Abutment to secure the immediate restoration, the accuracy should be sufficient for inserting a prefabricated final restoration at the time of implant surgery. However, no available CT-guided drill guide technology exists today with absolute precision. All articles on stereolithographic guides show error in all dimensions between virtual planning and obtained implant positions.[47] According to the literature, implants placed by bone-supported guides have the highest mean deviations, whereas implants placed by mucosa-supported guides have lower deviations.[48] Tooth-supported guides have the lowest measured deviation.[49] A single guide, using metal guide sleeves and rigid screw or pin fixation with specific drilling instrumentation, further minimizes error. Most systems use these fixation techniques to stabilize mucosal-supported guides.

The main advantage of inserting a final restoration immediately after implant placement is reduced treatment time. More commonly, clinicians who are using these technologies are placing temporary restorations after implant placement for many reasons. Regardless of whether a case is done flapless or not, there is no way to accurately predict the contours and anatomy of the healed gingiva, a significant issue for a laboratory technician fabricating a final restoration. Patients' esthetic demands can sometimes be great. Observation of the tissue response to the temporary restoration gives the restorative dentist invaluable information as to the gingival contours and esthetics required in preparation for the final restoration. In addition, regardless of whether an implant is placed guided or nonguided, a small number of implant failures occur. Typically, most surgery-related implant failures occur within the first 3 to 4 months after placement. Management of an implant failure, both surgically and restoratively, is best done before insertion of the final restoration. According to Abrahamsson and colleagues,[50] changing from a healing abutment to a permanent abutment did not result in a change in the dimension and quality of the transmucosal attachment that developed, and did not differ from the mucosal barrier that formed to a permanent abutment placed after surgery. In addition, an acrylic occlusal surface or a composite restoration has been found to have better shock absorbing behavior and reduces the force of occlusal effect compared with ceramic materials.[51] These are all valid reasons to place immediate acrylic temporary restorations, not immediate final porcelain restorations.

NobelGuide/NobelClinician (NobelBiocare) and Simplant (Materialise) are the 2 major systems currently in use. Clinically, the NobelGuide system is a more comprehensive system, with a full set of specific instrumentation for fully guided placement of NobelBiocare implants. NobelGuide is the only system currently available with the instrumentation for placement of tapered implants. The NobelGuide technology and instrumentation can be used for performing osteotomies for a straight-walled implant from any implant manufacturer. However, in these cases, the system can only be used for depth and direction of osteotomies. Because NobelGuide Implant Mounts are designed only for NobelBiocare implants, implants from other implant manufacturers cannot be accurately placed fully guided, through the guide. In these cases, the depth of implant placement should be evaluated with the guide off, usually after tissue flap elevation.

Simplant is designed as an open system for all implant systems. Although this feature increases its functionality, it is also a limitation because it is not perfectly adapted to 1 implant system in a comprehensive manner. Some clinicians believe that the Simplant software currently is more intuitive and easier to learn. Several implant manufacturers have recently developed and marketed instrumentation specific for the placement of straight-walled implants, flapless and fully guided, using the Simplant software (eg, Facilitate, AstraTech Dental; ExpertEase, Dentsply Friadent; Navigator, 3i/Biomet). Other manufacturers have developed nonstereolithographic model technologies for the fabrication of surgical guides (eg, IDent, Foster City, CA, USA; EZ Guide, Keystone Dental, Burlington, MA, USA; Straumann coDiagnostiX, Straumann, Basil, Switzerland) In these technologies, the surgical guide is created by scanning the patient while they are wearing a barium radiographic appliance, planning the implant placement virtually, then creating the surgical guide by milling the radiographic appliance according to the digital CT-based treatment plan. Guide sleeves are then added to the guide to aid in the depth and direction of osteotomies before implant placement.

The rationale for using minimally invasive procedures is to maximize patient comfort by minimizing traumatic injury to the tissues. Flapless insertion of dental implants has been found to have implant success rates comparable with conventional implant placement, also minimizing potential complications from soft tissue elevation such as infection, dehiscence, and soft and hard tissue necrosis.[30,52,53] Surgical guidance for drill depth and angulation, in combination with a flapless technique, minimizes the potential injury to underlying anatomic structures during the implant osteotomy preparation. Because fully guided instrumentation for implant insertion is not available in most Simplant cases, fully flapless surgery is not advised. Depth and angulation guidance of all osteotomies is possible, but accurate implant platform placement requires direct visualization of the bone, necessitating elevation of a flap. If using Navigator, ExpertEase, Facilitate, or Simplant fabricated NobelGuide compatible surgical guides, fully guided and flapless placement of implants is possible using available instrumentation.

CT-based technologies available today have limitations and questions that require further investigation as to their effect on guided surgery outcomes. The resolution and accuracy of specific CBCT machines compared with the gold standard of medical-grade CT scanners has been questioned.[54] NobelBiocare markets a calibration object that calibrates an individual CBCT/CT machine to an acrylic object of a known contour and density specifically for the NobelGuide protocol. Although theoretically the concept of a calibration object of this type makes sense, its efficacy is yet to be proved in the scientific literature.

The manufacture of a stereolithographic surgical guide or model involves reproducing the digitally planned dimensions of the surgical guide or model by using a laser beam to selectively solidify an ultraviolet-sensitive liquid resin. Stereolithographic materials have inherent potential problems that can lead to light sensitivity and expansion and/or shrinkage of the material. Leaving them exposed to light for extended periods of time, as well as sterilization in high-temperature autoclaves, distorts stereolithographic materials. The literature concludes that implant site preparation using surgical drill guides generates more heat than classic implant site preparation, regardless of the irrigation system used.[55]

SUMMARY

New technologies, based on 3D evaluation of patients for dental implants, has opened new avenues to clinicians for accurate and predictable diagnosis, planning, and treatment in a multidisciplinary patient-based approach. Communication between clinicians and understanding of these technologies are key components to improved case results and clinical outcomes. Analyzing, understanding, and adopting these technologies will open new doors for the dental team and benefit patients with more predictable outcomes.

The use of CT-guided implant planning and placement does not remove the need for the surgical and restorative team to diligently adhere to the basic principles of implant surgery and prosthetic dentistry. Well-established concepts of implant spacing, depth and angulation, case planning and engineering, minimally traumatic manipulation of soft and hard tissues, soft tissue and bone grafting, osseointegration healing time, soft and hard tissue healing, heat generation, dental materials, ideal occlusion, and many others must be maintained and adhered to. CT-guided implant surgery facilitates the placement of dental implants into an ideal position according to a restoratively driven treatment plan. The final tooth position is determined first. The ideal implant position is then planned, and the implant is then placed into that position with precision. Treatment plans should be created according to the requirements of an individual case and the comfort level of the surgical and restorative team. Cases can be treated with implants staged, with healing abutments, or immediately loaded with temporary, or in some circumstances, final restorations. Proper case selection and patient awareness, education, and compliance are all critical factors for success.

There is often a steep learning curve before there is successful incorporation of CT-guided surgery into a dental implant practice. Clinicians interested in these technologies are strongly encouraged to pursue continuing education. CT-guided implant surgery is not conventional implant surgery. Knowledge of CT scans, proprietary treatment planning software, the complete treatment protocols, and guided surgery instrumentation and surgical techniques, are all instrumental to a successful outcome. In addition, clinicians should take into consideration the inherent additional costs involved in the use of proprietary software and CAD/CAM processing technologies.

Of primary importance is good patient selection, in addition to appropriate diagnosis, planning and treatment. These requirements are best facilitated by a knowledge of CT-based technologies that enables the clinician to adhere to surgical, prosthetic, and biologic principles that will optimize patient care.

REFERENCES

1. Mozzo P, Procacci C, Tacconi A, et al. A new volumetric CT machine for dental imaging based on the cone beam technique: preliminary results. Eur Radiol 1998;8:1558.
2. Mah J, Hatcher D. Three dimensional craniofacial imaging. Am J Orthod Dentofacial Orthop 2004;126:308.
3. Hashimoto K, Yoshinori A, Kazui I, et al. A comparison of a new, limited cone beam computed tomography machine for dental use with a multi-detector row helical CT machine. Oral Surg Oral Med Oral Pathol Oral Radiol Endod 2005; 95:371.
4. Sukovic P. Cone beam computed tomography in craniofacial imaging. Orthod Craniofac Res 2003;6(Suppl 1):31.
5. Yu L, Vrieze TJ, Bruesewitz MR, et al. Dose and image quality evaluation of a dedicated cone-beam CT system for high-contrast neurologic applications. Am J Roentgenol 2010;194:W193.
6. Yamashina A, Tanimoto K, Sutthiprapaporn P, et al. The reliability of computed tomography (CT) values and dimensional measurements of the oropharyngeal region using cone beam CT: comparison with multidetector CT. Dentomaxillofac Radiol 2008;37:245.
7. Flicek K, Hara A, Silva A, et al. Reducing the radiation dose for CT colonography using adaptive statistical iterative reconstruction: a pilot study. Am J Roentgenol 2010;195:126–31.

8. Silva A, Lawder H, Hara A, et al. Innovations in CT dose reduction strategy: application of the adaptive statistical iterative reconstruction algorithm. Am J Roentgenol 2010;194:191–9.
9. Leipsic J, LaBounty T, Heilbron B, et al. Estimated radiation dose reduction using adaptive statistical iterative reconstruction in coronary CT angiography: the ERA-SIR study. Am J Roentgenol 2010;195:655–60.
10. Sagara Y, Hara A, Pavlicek W, et al. Abdominal CT: comparison of low-dose CT with adaptive statistical iterative reconstruction and routine-dose CT with filtered back projection in 53 patients. Am J Roentgenol 2010;195:713–9.
11. Liang X, Lambrichts I, Sun Y, et al. A comparative evaluation of cone beam computed tomography (CBCT) and multi-slice CT (MSCT). Part II: on 3D model accuracy. Eur J Radiol 2010;75:270–4.
12. Loubele M, Maes F, Schutyser F, et al. Assessment of bone segmentation quality of cone beam CT versus multislice spiral CT: a pilot study. Oral Surg Oral Med Oral Pathol Oral Radiol Endod 2006;102:225–34.
13. Rothman SL, Chaftez N, Rhodes ML, et al. CT in the preoperative assessment of the maxilla and mandible for endosseous implant surgery. Radiology 1988; 169(2):581.
14. Casselman JW, Deryckere F, Hermans R, et al. Denta Scan: CT software program used in the anatomic evaluation of the mandible and maxilla in the perspective of endosseous implant surgery. Rofo 1991;155(1):4–10.
15. Villari N, Fanfani F. Diagnostic contribution of CT in implantology: use of a new Denta-Scan reconstruction program. Radiol Med 1992;83(5):608–14.
16. Tal H, Moses O. A comparison of panoramic radiography with computed tomography in the planning of implant surgery. Dentomaxillofac Radiol 1991;20(1):40–2.
17. Available at: http://sites.google.com/site/simplantisrael/simplantsources. Web history-about CSI. Accessed January, 2011.
18. Ramez J, Donazzan M, Chanavaz M, et al. The contribution of scanner imagery in implant surgery and sinus overflow using frontal oblique orthogonal reconstruction. Rev Stomatol Chir Maxillofac 1992;93:212–4.
19. Pattijn V, van Cleynenbreugel T, vander Sloten J, et al. Structural and radiological parameters for the nondestructive characterization of trabecular bone. Ann Biomed Eng 2001;29:1064–73.
20. Sonick M, Abrahams J, Faiella R. A comparison of the accuracy of periapical, panoramic, and computerized tomographic radiographs in locating the mandibular canal. Int J Oral Maxillofac Implants 1994;9(4):455–60.
21. Todd A, Gher M, Quintero G, et al. Interpretation of linear and computed tomograms in the assessment of implant recipient sites. J Periodontol 1993;64:1243–9.
22. Gehr ME, Richardson AC. The accuracy of dental radiographic techniques used for evaluation of implant fixture placement. Int J Periodontics Restorative Dent 1995;15:268–83.
23. van Steenberghe D, Glauser R, Blombäck U, et al. A computed tomographic scan derived customized surgical template and fixed prosthesis for flapless surgery and immediate loading of implants in fully edentulous maxillae. A prospective multicenter study. Clin Implant Dent Relat Res 2005;7(Suppl 1): S111–20.
24. Tardieu P, Vrielinck L. Implantologie assistèe par ordinateur: le propramme SimPlant/SurgiCase et le SAFE System mis en charge immediate d'unbridge mandibulaire avec des impalt transmuqueux. Implant 2003;9:15–28 [in French].
25. Rosenfeld AL, Mandelaris GA, Tardieu PB. Prosthetically directed implant placement using computer software to ensure precise placement and predictable

prosthetic outcomes. Part 3: stereolithographic drilling guides that do not require bone exposure and the immediate delivery of teeth. Int J Periodontics Restorative Dent 2006;26:493.

26. Vrielinck L, Politis C, Schepers S, et al. Image-based planning and clinical validation of zygoma and pterygoid implant placement in patients with severe bone atrophy using customized drill guides. Preliminary results from a prospective clinical follow-up study. Int. J Oral Maxillofac Surg 2003;32:7–14.

27. Sarment DP, Sukovic P, Clinthorne N. Accuracy of implant placement with a stereolithographic surgical guide. Int J Oral Maxillofac Implants 2003;18:571–7.

28. Hahn J. Single stage, immediate loading, and flapless surgery. J Oral Implantol 2000;26:193–8.

29. Campelo LD, Dominguez Camara JR. Flapless implant surgery: a 10 year clinical retrospective analysis. Int J Oral Maxillofac Implants 2002;17:271–6.

30. Becker W, Goldstein M, Becker BE, et al. Minimally invasive flapless implant surgery: a prospective multicenter study. Clin Implant Dent Relat Res 2005; 7(Suppl 1):S21–7.

31. Becker W, Wikesjo UME, Sennerby L, et al. Histologic evaluation of implants following flapless and flapped surgery: a study in canines. J Periodontol 2006; 77:1717–22.

32. Abboud M, Wahl G. Clinical benefits, risks, accuracy of cone beam CT based guided implant placement. Clin Oral Implants Res 2009;20:909.

33. Johansson B, Grepe A, Wannfors K, et al. A clinical study of changes in the volume of bone grafts in the atrophic maxilla. Dentomaxillofac Radiol 2001; 30(3):157–61.

34. Verhoeven JW, Ruijter J, Cune MS, et al. Onlay grafts in combination with endosseous implants in severe mandibular atrophy; one year results of a prospective, quantitative radiological study. Clin Oral Implants Res 2000;11(6):583–94.

35. Smolka W, Eggensperger N, Carollo V, et al. Changes in the volume and density of calvarial split bone grafts after alveolar ridge augmentation. Clin Oral Implants Res 2006;17(2):149–55.

36. Krennmair G, Krainhofner M, Maier H, et al. Computerized tomography-assisted calculation of sinus augmentation volume. Int J Oral Maxillofac Implants 2005; 21(6):907–13.

37. Orentlicher GP, Goldsmith DH, Horowitz AD. Applications of 3-dimensional virtual computerized tomography technology in oral and maxillofacial surgery: current therapy. J Oral Maxillofac Surg 2010;68:1933–59.

38. Marx RE. Osteoradionecrosis: a new concept of its pathophysiology. J Oral Maxillofac Surg 1983;41:283.

39. Marx RE, Ames JR. The use of hyperbaric oxygen therapy in bony reconstruction of the irradiated and tissue-deficient patient. J Oral Maxillofac Surg 1982;40:412–20.

40. Granstrom G. Placement of dental implants in irradiated bone: The case for using hyperbaric oxygen. J Oral Maxillofac Surg 2006;64:812–8.

41. Granstrom G. Radiotherapy, osseointegration, and hyperbaric oxygen therapy. Periodontol 2000 2003;33:245.

42. Koga DH, Salvajoli JV, Alves FA. Dental extractions and radiotherapy in head and neck oncology: review of the literature. Oral Dis 2008;14:40–4.

43. Horowitz AD, Orentlicher GP, Goldsmith DH. Case report- computerized implantology: for the irradiated patient. J Oral Maxillofac Surg 2009;67:619–23.

44. Komiyama A, Pettersson A, Hultin M, et al. Virtually planned and template-guided implant surgery: an experimental model matching approach. Clin Oral Implants Res 2010;22:308–13.

45. Wagner A, Wanschitz F, Birkfellner W, et al. Computer-aided placement of endosseous oral implants in patients after ablative tumour surgery: assessment of accuracy. Clin Oral Implants Res 2003;14:340–8.
46. Casap N, Tarazi E, Wexler A, et al. Intraoperative computerized navigation for flapless implant surgery and immediate loading in the edentulous mandible. Int J Oral Maxillofac Implants 2005;20:92–8.
47. D'Haese J, Van De Velde T, Komiyama A, et al. Accuracy and complications using computer-designed stereolithographic surgical guides for oral rehabilitation by means of dental implants: a review of the literature. Clin Implant Dent Relat Res 2010. [Epub ahead of print]. DOI:10.1111/j.1708-8208.2010.00275.x.
48. Arisan V, Karabuda ZC, Ozdemir T. Accuracy of two stereolithographic guide systems for computer-aided implant placement: a computed tomography-based clinical comparative study. J Periodontol 2010;81:43–51.
49. Ozan O, Turkyilmaz I, Ersoy AE, et al. Clinical accuracy of 3 different types of computed tomography-derived stereolithographic surgical guides in implant placement. J Oral Maxillofac Surg 2009;67:394–401.
50. Abrahamsson I, Berglundh T, Sekino S, et al. Tissue reactions to abutment shift: an experimental study in dogs. Clin Implant Dent Relat Res 2003;5:82–8.
51. Gracis SE, Nicholls JI, Chalupnik JD, et al. Shock-absorbing behavior of five restorative materials used on implants. Int J Prosthodont 1991;4:282–91.
52. Arisan V, Karabuda CZ, Ozdemir T. Implant surgery using bone- and mucosa-supported stereolithographic guides in totally edentulous jaws: surgical and post-operative outcomes of computer-aided vs. standard techniques. Clin Oral Implants Res 2010;21:980–8.
53. Cannizzaro G, Torchio C, Leone M, et al. Immediate versus early loading of flapless-placed implants supporting maxillary full-arch prostheses: a randomised controlled clinical trial. Eur J Oral Implantol 2008;1:127–39.
54. Van Assche N, van Steenberghe D, Guerrero ME, et al. Accuracy of implant placement based on pre-surgical planning of three-dimensional cone-beam images: a pilot study. J Clin Periodontol 2007;34:816–21.
55. Misir AF, Sumer M, Yenisey M, et al. Effect of surgical drill guide on heat generated from implant drilling. J Oral Maxillofac Surg 2009;67:2663–8.

Rescue Implant Concept: The Expanded Use of the Zygoma Implant in the Graftless Solutions

Edmond Bedrossian, DDS*

KEYWORDS

- Zygomatic implant • Rescue implant • Dental implants
- Edentulous maxilla

The use of tilted implants in a graftless approach for immediate loading has been well documented in the literature. This treatment for fully edentulous and often times highly resorbed maxillae allows for rehabilitation with a fixed prosthesis. The purpose of this article is to describe criteria for use of the zygomatic implant, including the expanded use of the zygoma implant in cases where failure of one of the anteriorly or posteriorly tilted implants has occurred in All-on-Four treatment. Zygomatic implant placement becomes a rescue procedure, which allows for continuity of care without resorting to a removable denture.

The treatment of the edentulous maxilla using dental implants has been evolving in the last decade. The edentulous maxilla presents with unique anatomic considerations. The presence of the maxillary sinus limits the volume of the available bone for placement of implants. Because of this, implants are restricted to the premaxilla unless grafting is preformed, which commonly results in a tissue-borne overdenture appliance.[1]

Because of a desire to maintain bone through "internal loading", bone-grafting procedures for implant placement have been advocated to biomechanically stimulate the entire maxilla via anteroposterior distribution of implants.[2–6] But to avoid grafting procedures and transitional dentures, the concept of tilting implants was developed to achieve immediate function. This idea of implant tilting moves the prosthetic support posteriorly (**Fig. 1**).[7–9] Concern about increased "bending moments" (unfavorable

This article was previously published in the May 2011 issue of *Oral and Maxillofacial Surgery Clinics of North America*.
Department of Oral & Maxillofacial Residency Training Program, Dugoni School of Dentisty, San Francisco, CA, USA
* 450 Sutter Street, Suite 2439, San Francisco, CA 94108.
E-mail address: oms@sfimplants.com

Dent Clin N Am 55 (2011) 745–777
doi:10.1016/j.cden.2011.07.009
0011-8532/11/$ – see front matter © 2011 Elsevier Inc. All rights reserved.

dental.theclinics.com

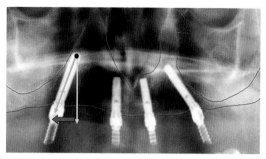

Fig. 1. By tilting the platform of the distal implant, greater anterior-posterior length is achieved.

lateral forces) from tilted implants has not been demonstrated because posterior cantilevers are less than for axial placement and immediate cross-arch stabilization is used.[8]

In cases where only premaxillary alveolar bone remains, the placement of zygomatic implants, used in a staged fashion, well establishes posterior support.[10–15] But now, recent studies have shown favorable outcomes using *zygomatic implants and immediate loading* with fixed provisional prostheses.[13,16–18]

In review of the literature, the longest-term study followed a 2-stage protocol. In 2004 Branemark and colleagues[14] reported a cumulative survival rate (CSR) of 94.2% on a 5- to 10-year follow-up of 28 subjects using 52 zygoma implants. In a recent prospective study by Bedrossian,[19] a CSR of 97.2% was observed following 36 subjects having received 74 zygoma implants over a 7-year period.

PATIENT SELECTION

A systematic preoperative evaluation of patients is required before surgical treatment. Both surgical and prosthetic needs must be considered for a predictable outcome. The preoperative evaluation takes into consideration available alveolar bone in the different zones of the maxilla (**Fig. 2**) and the presence or lack of a composite defect. This evaluation then determines whether the final prosthesis is a ceramo-metal bridge or profile prosthesis. Treatment is prescribed based on the availability of bone in maxillary zones. Zone I is the premaxilla, zone II is the bicuspid zone, and zone III is the posterior maxilla. An anterior tilted implant concept is considered in patients

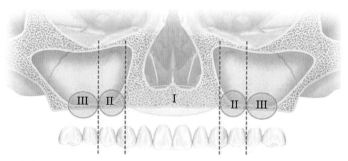

Fig. 2. Zones of the maxilla; presence or absence of the zones dictates the surgical concept.

with bone in both zone I and II. The zygomatic implant concept is considered in patients who demonstrate bone in zone I only (**Table 1**).

Evaluation of the esthetics of the final prosthesis is made by recognizing the transition line between the prosthesis and the residual edentulous crestal soft tissues. The transition line must be apical to the smile line for a favorable outcome.[16]

RADIOGRAPHIC EVALUATION

Although computerized and conventional tomography can be used, the panorex radiograph is critical in the initial evaluation of patients.[12–14] The presence of alveolar bone in the premaxilla (zone I) and the lack of bone in the bicuspid and the molar regions, zones II and III respectively, are the main indications for considering the zygomatic concept. Axial CT scans can be obtained to further evaluate the maxillary sinus. The width of the residual alveolar bone as well as the width and height of the zygomatic body can be visualized in frontal reformatted sections of axial CT images.

Further evaluation of the zygomatic bone has also been described.[20] Although not absolutely necessary, reformatted frontal images in 2-to 3-mm cuts afford the less experienced operator more information for planning surgery (**Fig. 3**). The sagittal view of a 3-dimentional radiograph also provides information as to the anteroposterior dimension of the zygoma (**Fig. 4**). The presence of sinus pathology, including but not limited to the thickening of the sinus membrane, may be ruled out in both the panorex as well as tomographic studies.

SURGICAL PROTOCOL

The surgical procedure begins by making a crestal incision across the edentulous arch. Bilateral releasing incisions are made over the maxillary tuberosities. A vertical window is made on the lateral wall of the maxilla paralleling the junction of the posterior aspect of the lateral maxillary wall and the lateral aspect of the posterior maxillary wall accessing the sinus (**Fig. 5**). The sinus membrane may be removed or reflected inside of the lateral wall of the maxillary sinus. It is critical to be aware of the position of the sinus membrane and to ensure that it does not attach to the zygomatic implant during insertion because introduction of soft tissue into the body of the zygoma will lead to nonosseointegration.

The osteotomy is initiated by the use of a round bur followed by a 2.9-mm twist drill. A 2.9- to 3.5-mm pilot drill stabilizes the 3.5-mm drill, which completes the osteotomy both at the maxillary crest as well as the body of the zygoma (**Fig. 6**). If greater than 3 mm of crestal bone is identified, the alveolar portion of the osteotomy is completed by introduction of the 4.0-mm twist drill. In cases where there is a limited crestal bone width or height, the 4.0-mm drill is not used. Prior to implant placement, and at all

Table 1
Treatment concept recommendations based on the presence of alveolar bone in different zones of the maxilla

Presence of Bone	Surgical Approach
Zone I, II, III	Traditional (axial)
Zone I, II	All-on-Four
Zone I only	Zygomatic implants
Insufficient bone	Quad zygoma

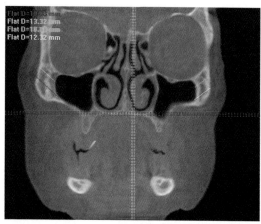

Fig. 3. Frontal cone beam computer tomography (CBCT) view of the maxillary sinuses and the body of the zygomatic bone.

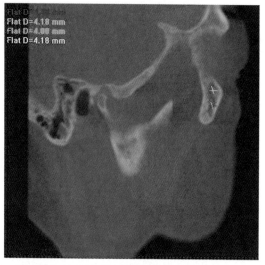

Fig. 4. Sagittal (lateral cephalometric) view of the left zygoma.

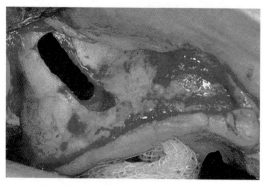

Fig. 5. Axis opening into the right maxillary sinus.

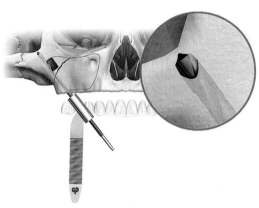

Fig. 6. The tip of the drill exits the lateral boney wall of the zygoma during preparation of the osteotomy; hence a quad-cortically stabilized implant site.

times during preparation of the osteotomy, the entire surgical path of the drill is visualized.[12,17]

The 45° angulation of the zygomaticus implant allows for the platform of the implant to be on the same plane as vertically placed implants in the premaxilla. To facilitate implant placement, a premounted implant carrier allows for ease of handling despite using a straight hand piece. To ensure proper orientation, the long axis of the screwdriver shaft is placed into the screw that secures the implant carrier (**Fig. 7**). The shaft of this screwdriver must be at right angles to the edentulous ridge to ensure proper orientation.

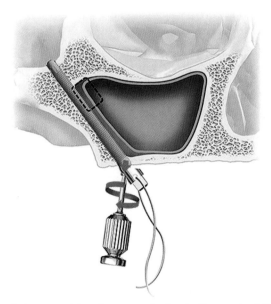

Fig. 7. The shaft of the screwdriver is perpendicular to the crest of the maxillary ridge placing the implant platform in the correct relationship to the alveolar crest.

A minimum of 2 premaxillary implants and 2 zygoma implants are used.[21] The use of 4 implants distributed along the maxillary arch and cross arch splinted has been documented by Branemark and Skalak[22] as biomechanically stable (**Fig. 8**). When immediate loading is considered, a double-threaded implant, (Nobel Speedy, Nobel Biocare, Gothenburg, Sweden) has been used. The zygomatic implant is an external hex implant. Because of this external hex, premaxillary implants are recommended to maintain uniformity during the restorative phase. All premaxillary implants are placed with an initial insertion torque setting of 20 Ncm. Upon stalling of the hand piece, the insertion torque is increased to 40 Ncm allowing complete insertion and seating of the implants. Hand insertion is used in cases where the hand piece stalls at the 40 Ncm setting. The zygomatic implant is hand driven to its final insertion depth until the implant platform is intimately in contact with the lateral wall of the maxillary alveolus. The criteria for the immediate loading of the premaxillary implants as well as the zygoma implants include a minimum of 40 Ncm of insertion torque.[16]

In patients who receive immediate provisional fixed prostheses, 3-0 gut is used to close the wound and the existing full denture is converted to an immediate provisional by use of multiunit abutments and titanium temporary cylinders.[16,19]

After placement a 6-month osseointegration period is allowed before phase II. At phase II the provisional prosthesis is removed and abutment screws retorqued. The lack of implant sensitivity renders the implants osseointegrated.

On occasion, if an implant rotates along its axis at stage II evaluation, it is deemed failed and should be removed.

Prior to the removal of a failed implant, one that is supporting a fixed appliance, a decision has to be made for replacement. Most patients will not consent to the use of a transitional denture while the failed site heals in preparation for replacement. Therefore, the surgeon has to consider the possibility of removal of the failed implant and immediate replacement with reattachment of the provisional prosthesis. In these cases, consideration for placement of a zygomatic implant as a rescue implant should strongly be considered. Four clinical case presentations are discussed:

1. Management of a failed zygomatic implant
2. Intraoperative management of an "anterior tilted" implant with inadequate initial stability
3. Management of a failed "anterior tilted" implant
4. Management of a failed premaxillary implant.

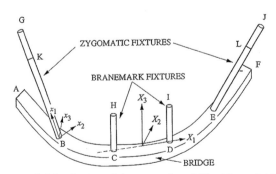

Fig. 8. Skalak-Branemark 4 implant model cross arch stabilized by a rigid prosthesis.

CLINICAL PRESENTATION 1

In cases where a zygomatic implant has failed and there is a lack of alveolar bone and patients are unwilling to use a removable appliance, clinicians are faced with a difficult dilemma. The author has experienced 2 such cases, both presenting with the failure of a single zygomatic implant. In one case, 6 months after immediate loading, the patient was seen for phase II. The patient presented with a stable provisional prosthesis, but when the prosthesis was removed the zygomatic implant rotated. The patient was informed of this finding and a surgical plan for replacement was scheduled.

In the following case studies, the immediate placement of a new zygoma implant is described following the removal of a failed zygoma implant.

A 65-year-old patient presented with a maxillary denture that she did not wear because of instability. The clinical examination was consistent with a moderately resorbed maxillary arch (**Fig. 9**). The radiographic examination demonstrated the presence of bone in zone I only (**Fig. 10**). Therefore, a treatment was planned for the patient to receive 2 premaxillary implants as well as 2 zygomatic implants (**Fig. 11**). After placement of the implants, the soft tissues were closed in preparation for the conversion of the patient's denture into provisional immediate load prosthesis. The 1-month postoperative visit was uneventful and the patient presented with a stable provisional prosthesis.

At the sixth month phase II appointment the maxillary provisional prosthesis was stable with bilateral equal occlusal contacts (**Fig. 12**). However, upon removal of the prosthesis the right zygomatic implant was found to be mobile (**Fig. 13**).

Mobility of the zygomatic implant horizontally does not indicate failure or the lack of osseointegration because there is generally a lack of supporting alveolar bone, often only 0 to 3 mm in the premolar-molar region. Therefore, resorption of this limited amount of bone may lead to mesiodistal and or buccal-palatal motion of the crestal portion of the implant, which does not indicate failure. However, the implant must not rotate on its axis. The stability of the zygomatic implant is at the apex, within the body of the zygomatic bone. Therefore, upon torqueing of the zygoma implant abutment, if rotation is observed, the implant has failed and needs to be removed and replaced.

Three-dimensional radiographic evaluation of the right zygomatic implant suggested the lack of osseointegration secondary to the presence of radiolucency around

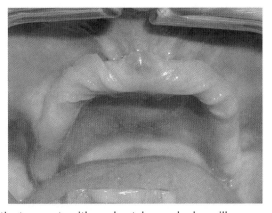

Fig. 9. Female patient presents with moderately resorbed maxilla.

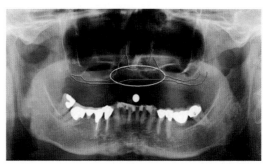

Fig. 10. Evaluation of the zones of the maxilla is consistent with presence of zone I only.

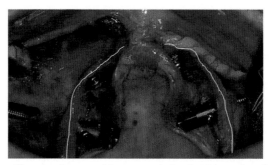

Fig. 11. Two premaxillary implants and 2 zygomatic implants are placed.

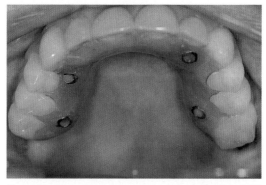

Fig. 12. During the 6 months of osseointegration period, the patient did not experience any adverse reaction.

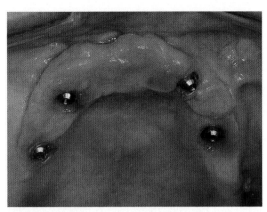

Fig. 13. Implant number 3 rotated on its axis when 35 Ncm of torque was applied to the abutment screw.

the apical portion of the implant. The radiographic appearance, along with the presence of rotational mobility, confirmed the lack of osseointegration.

Further radiographic evaluation demonstrated availability of bone superior to the existing zygoma implant (**Fig. 14**). The surgical plan was removal of the failed implant and using the same entry point to replace the existing implant.

The patient was sedated and a localized flap was made to expose the posterior lateral maxilla. Upon reflection of the flap, it was observed that the previous boney window was covered by a moderately thick soft tissue (**Fig. 15**). After removing the membrane coverage of the sinus window, the failed implant was rotated out without difficulty and a new zygomatic implant placed into position (**Fig. 16**). A resorbable membrane was secured at the alveolar crest using mini titanium screws. (The purpose of the membrane is to create a floor for the leading edge of the flaps to rest over as the surgical wound is healing. This technique (**Fig. 17**) limits the potential for the formation of an oral-antral communication.) The flap was then sutured around the abutment and immediate load provisional placed. The postoperative panorex demonstrated the position of the implants and the stabilized membrane (**Fig. 18**).

In preparation for the reconnection of the provisional prosthesis, the existing temporary titanium cylinder was trephined out from the provisional. The provisional was then secured to 3 osseointegrated implants (**Fig. 19**). A new titanium cylinder was attached

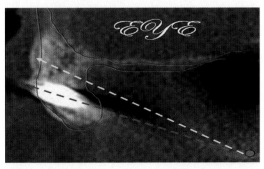

Fig. 14. Trajectory of the new implant compared with the trajectory of the existing failed implant.

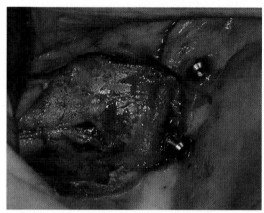

Fig. 15. Partial flap exposing the right posterior lateral maxilla.

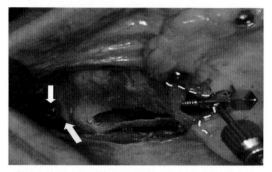

Fig. 16. Placement of the new zygoma implant.

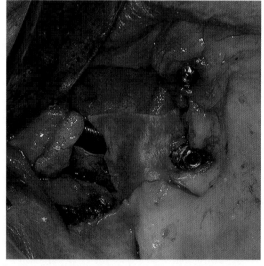

Fig. 17. Fixation of a resorbable membrane over the alveolar defect.

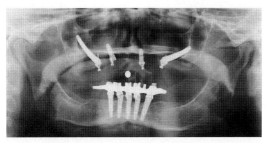

Fig. 18. Immediate panorex of the replacement of the right zygoma implant.

to the new implant abutment (**Fig. 20**) and intraorally luted to the remaining prosthesis. Upon completion of the connection, the patient was discharged (**Fig. 21**). After an additional 6 months time, the provisional prosthesis was removed and all implants were found to be stable. The final metal-based prosthesis was fabricated (**Fig. 22**). The patient was extremely satisfied with the esthetics and function.

The ability to immediately replace the zygomatic implant and reconnect the provisional prosthesis at the same time is a tremendous service for this group of patients.

CLINICAL PRESENTATION 2

The immediate loading of implants is in part dependent on achieving 40 Ncm of insertion torque at the time of implant placement. In cases where 40 Ncm has not been obtained, immediate loading is not indicated. The following case illustrates the management of a clinical presentation that had poor initial stability, leading to aborting the intended immediate loading. However, by using the zygoma implant as a rescue implant, management of this condition was possible.

A 45-year-old female patient presented with failing dentition of her partially edentulous maxilla. She had resisted any form of treatment that would entail the use of a transitional full-maxillary denture (**Fig. 23**). She presented with multiple missing teeth and failing remaining teeth (**Fig. 24**). She had a partially visible transition line (**Fig. 25**).

Clinical Evaluation
1. Composite defect: present
2. Final prosthetic design: fixed profile prosthesis

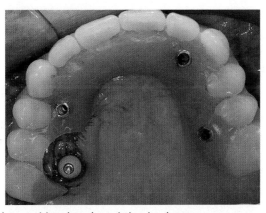

Fig. 19. Securing the provisional to the existing implants.

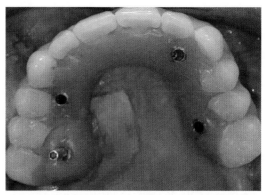

Fig. 20. Luting the new temporary titanium cylinder to the provisional.

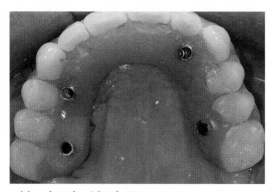

Fig. 21. Secured provisional to the 4 implants.

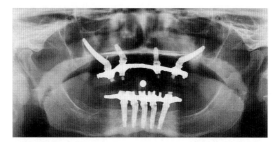

Fig. 22. Final panoramic radiograph.

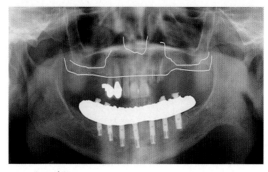

Fig. 23. Available zones I and II.

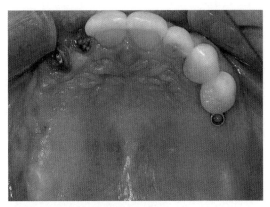

Fig. 24. Nonrestorable remaining maxillary teeth.

3. Transition line: visible
4. Zones of the maxilla: presence of I and II
5. Surgical concept: anterior tilted concept.

Treatment Plan
1. Removal of the existing maxillary dentition
2. Alveoloplasty to move the final transition line apically
3. Placement of 2 axial and 2 tilted implants
4. Immediate loading by conversion of an immediate full maxillary denture if 40 Ncm insertion torque was attained.

TREATMENT

Reflection of a full-thickness flap exposed the remaining teeth and the alveolar housing. Careful removal of the teeth and alveoloplasty was performed in preparation for placement of the implants (**Figs. 26** and **27**). Tilted implants were planned for the posterior maxilla and 2 axial implants for the premaxilla. For the right posterior, a 2-mm osteotomy was made and the relationship of the 2-mm drill to the anterior wall of the maxilla was evaluated using digital radiography (**Figs. 28** and **29**). Upon completion of the osteotomy, the implant was placed. A 30, multiunit abutment was secured

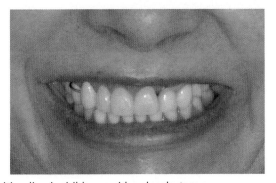

Fig. 25. The transition line is visible; consider alveolectomy.

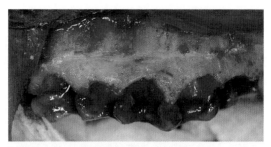

Fig. 26. Removal of the anterior maxillary teeth.

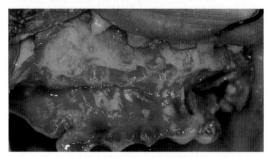

Fig. 27. Alveolectomy moving the transition line apically.

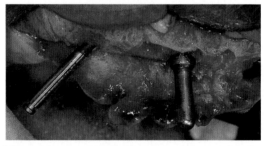

Fig. 28. Anterior tilting of the posterior implant in position number 3.

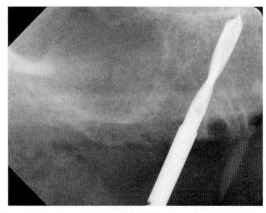

Fig. 29. Confirmation of the angulation of the tilted implant using the 2-mm drill.

(**Fig. 30**). Upon torqueing at 20 Ncm, slight rotation of the implant was observed. At this time several decisions are available for the surgeon:

1. Leave the existing implant alone and DO NOT immediately load.
2. Remove the implant and attempt achieving 40 Ncm with a longer implant of the same platform.
3. Remove the implant and place a wide diameter Nobel Active (Nobel Biocare, Gothenburg, Sweden) implant because it has a regular platform prosthetic table and will accept a 30angulated abutment.
4. Remove the implant and place a zygomatic implant.

The decision in this case was to remove the implant and place a zygomatic implant, which demonstrated 40 Ncm plus insertion torque.

After 6 months of osseointegration, the provisional prosthesis was removed and the 35 Ncm of torque was reapplied to the straight, multiunit abutments and 20 Ncm of torque to the angulated abutment to confirm osseointegration before impression and fabrication of the final profile prosthesis (**Fig. 31**).

CLINICAL PRESENTATION 3

In cases where failure of a distal implant occurs during the 6-month osseointegration period, the zygoma implant may be considered for continuation of the use of the immediate load prosthesis.

A 72-year-old man with failing remaining maxillary dentition was seeking a fixed prosthesis. The remaining anterior maxillary teeth were mobile, having supported a partial denture for 15 years. The following clinical evaluation and treatment plan was considered.

Clinical Evaluation
1. Composite defect: present (minimal)
2. Final prosthetic design: fixed profile prosthesis
3. Transition line: not visible
4. Zones of the maxilla: presence of zones I and II bilaterally (**Fig. 32**)
5. Surgical concept: anterior tilted concept.

Treatment Plan
1. Removal of the existing maxillary dentition
2. Placement of 2 axial and 2 tilted implants (anterior tilted concept)

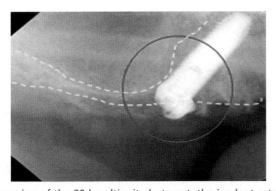

Fig. 30. Upon torqueing of the 30 I multiunit abutment, the implant rotated at 20 Ncm.

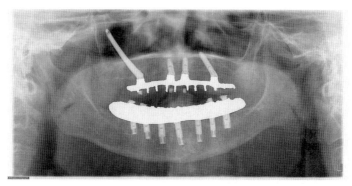

Fig. 31. Final panorex with the completed fixed implant prosthesis.

3. Immediate loading by conversion of the immediate full maxillary denture (if 40 Ncm insertion torque).

The patient was sedated, the remaining maxillary teeth removed, and implants placed (**Fig. 33**). The maxillary provisional prosthesis was immediately connected to the newly placed implants with bilateral equal occlusion and excellent esthetics (**Fig. 34**).

Three months after the surgical procedure, the patient presented with a missing portion of the maxillary prosthesis (**Fig. 35**). The radiograph demonstrated the missing abutment and associated temporary titanium cylinder. Upon interviewing the patient, he stated that the prosthesis had been loose for more than 1 week, with its eventual fracture and separation from the rest of the prosthesis.

After evaluation of the patient, the decision to replace the implant was made. The various surgical options available are the following:

1. Remove the implant and attempt to achieve 40 Ncm with a longer implant of the same platform.
2. Remove the implant and place a wide-diameter implant.
3. Remove the implant and place a zygomatic implant and immediately load the patient.

TREATMENT

A full-thickness mucoperiosteal flap was developed over the right posterior maxillary implant. The implant was removed (**Fig. 36**) revealing a large crestal defect (**Fig. 37**).

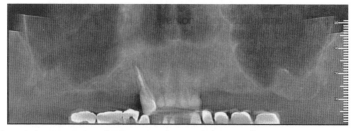

Fig. 32. Remaining zones I and II boney volume of the maxilla.

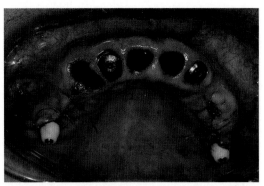

Fig. 33. Flapless approach to removal of the teeth and placement of the implants.

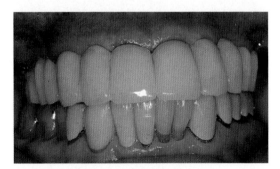

Fig. 34. Stable occlusion with the provisional prosthesis.

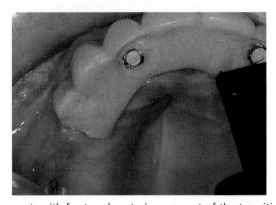

Fig. 35. Patient presents with fractured posterior segment of the transitional appliance.

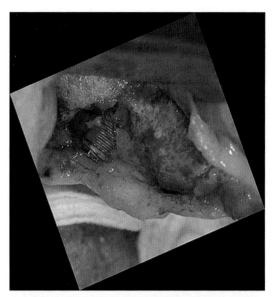

Fig. 36. Debridement of the soft tissues from the buccal aspect of the mobile implant.

Because of the loss of the buccal plate, the decision to place a zygoma implant was made (**Fig. 38**).

The palatal of the zygoma implant platform was stabilized against the remaining edge of the hard palate (**Fig. 39**). To minimize the potential for the formation of an

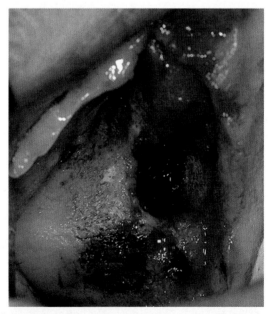

Fig. 37. Boney defect evident after removal of the implant and debridement of the implant site.

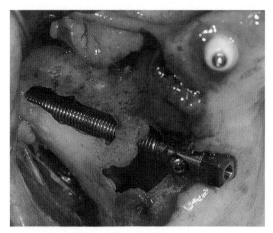

Fig. 38. Placement of an immediate zygoma implant.

oral antral communication over the existing crestal boney defect, a resorbable membrane was secured to the newly placed zygoma implant by stabilizing it to the implant platform by the multiunit abutment and to the maxillary wall using mini titanium screws (**Figs. 40** and **41**).

The temporary titanium cylinder was removed from the fractured portion of the provisional prosthesis. The fractured portion was luted into place capturing the position of the newly placed implant. Six months of healing time was allowed (**Fig. 42**) before the final profile prosthesis was placed (**Figs. 43** and **44**).

CLINICAL PRESENTATION 4

In cases where failure of the premaxillary (anterior) implant occurs during the six month osseointegration period and there is lack of remaining alveolar bone in Zone I, the zygoma implant may be considered for continuation of the use of the immediate load prosthesis.

A 70 year old male patient presents with failing of his remaining maxillary dentition. Due to the presence of an unrepaired left maxillary alveolar cleft in the cuspid region, a significant lack of anterior-posterior development of his maxilla is present leading to a pseudo-Class III appearance (**Fig. 45**). His panoramic radiograph demonstrated

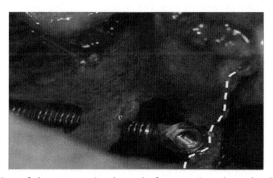

Fig. 39. Stabilization of the zygoma implant platform against the palatal bone.

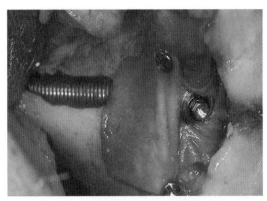

Fig. 40. Stabilization of the apical portion of the membrane by 1.5-mm titanium screws.

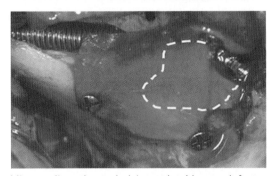

Fig. 41. The dotted line outlines the underlying palatal boney defect.

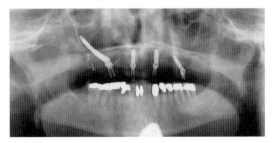

Fig. 42. Immediate postoperative radiograph.

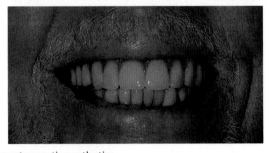

Fig. 43. Excellent postoperative esthetics.

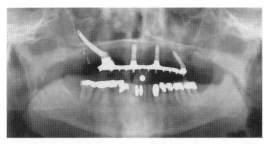

Fig. 44. Final panorex with complete seating of all components.

limited posterior maxillary alveolar bone for the placement of implants (**Fig. 46**). Clinical and radiographic examination revealed the following findings:

Clinical Evaluation
1. Composite defect: present
2. Final prosthetic design: fixed profile prosthesis
3. Transition line: not visible
4. Zones of the maxilla: after removal of the remaining maxillary teeth, presence of zone I only remains
5. Surgical concept: posterior tilted (Zygoma) concept.

Treatment Plan
1. Removal of the existing maxillary dentition
2. Surgical technique: zygoma concept
3. Immediate loading by conversion of the immediate full maxillary denture, if 40 Ncm insertion torque is attained.

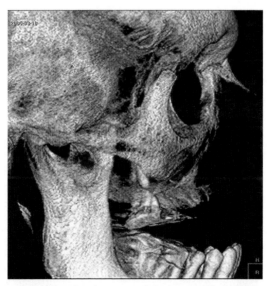

Fig. 45. Lack of anteroposterior development of the premaxilla in the patient with alveolar cleft.

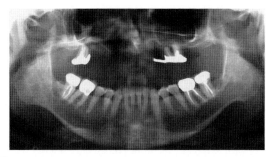

Fig. 46. Preoperative panorex.

TREATMENT

Two axial implants, a right anterior tilted and a left posterior tilted implant was placed after removal of the existing teeth without complication (**Fig. 47**) and the implants were immediately loaded (**Fig. 48**) by converting a new full denture fabricated earlier. After 3 months the patient presented with pain in the left axial implant (**Fig. 49**). After removal of the prosthesis, implant no 12 was deemed failed and was removed. A new implant was immediately placed in position no 10 (**Fig. 50**), the existing temporary titanium cylinder in position 12 was trephined out and the new position of the implant no 10 was captured and incorporated into the immediate load prosthesis (**Fig. 51**). Radiographic presentation of the original position of implant no 10 and the new position of the left axial implant is demonstrated in the **Figs. 52** and **53** respectively.

After 14 weeks, implant no 10 became sensitive and was removed leaving the patient with 3 osseointegrated implants (**Fig. 54**). The presence of limited bone quality and quantity in the left maxillary alveolar cleft region is suspected as the reason for the loss of the 2 left maxillary axial implants. The existing number and distribution of implants was not viewed as a good long-term solution. Therefore, the following treatment options were considered.

1. No further treatment, connection of the implants by a bar and fabrication of an implant retained maxillary overdenture
2. Using autogenous cortico-cancelous or an allograft material to reconstruct the left maxillary alveolar cleft in the area 9 through 12
3. Consideration for the placement of a second zygomatic implant in the left zygoma above the existing zygomatic implant.

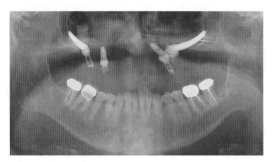

Fig. 47. Immediate postoperative panorex.

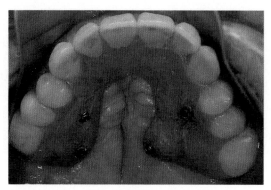

Fig. 48. Immediate load provisional prosthesis.

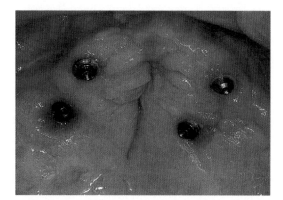

Fig. 49. Implant number 12 demonstrated mobility during the osseointegration period.

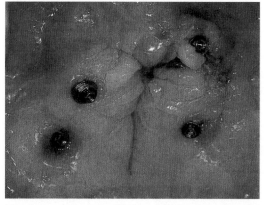

Fig. 50. Removal of implant number 12 with immediate placement of implant number 10.

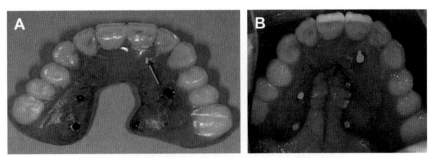

Fig. 51. (A) Removal of the existing titanium cylinder from positions number 12. (B) Immediate connection of newly placed implant number 10 to the provisional prosthesis.

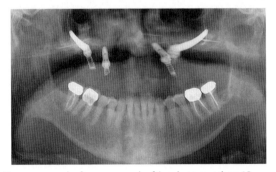

Fig. 52. Preoperative panorex before removal of implant number 12.

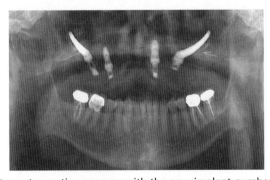

Fig. 53. Immediate postoperative panorex with the new implant number 10.

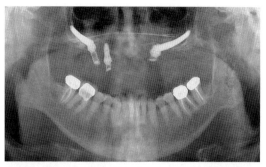

Fig. 54. Panorex demonstration the failed implant no 10 three months after its placement.

After a 3-dimentional radiographs was obtained, the left zygoma was studied to see the feasibility for the placement of a second zygoma implant as the patient did not want to have a final removable appliance nor undergo extensive bone grafting procedure (**Fig. 55**). The dry skull model in **Fig. 56** demonstrates the position of two zygomatic implants within the body of one zygomatic bone. The superior implant within the zygoma exits the anterior portion of the maxillary alveolus and the inferior implant exits more posteriorly in the traditional position within the alveolar ridge.

Following the aforementioned principles, a second implant was placed superior to the existing zygomatic implant which exited in the cuspid region of the alveolar ridge (**Fig. 57**). The immediate load provisional prosthesis was modified and connected to all implants .

The postoperative 3-dimentional radiographic studies were consistent with achieving the intended implant positions (**Figs. 58** and **59**). After 6 months of osseointegration for the newly placed zygoma implant, the provisional prosthesis was removed (**Fig. 60**), all implants were stable. The final profile prosthesis was fabricated with stable function and good esthetics (**Figs. 61** and **62**).

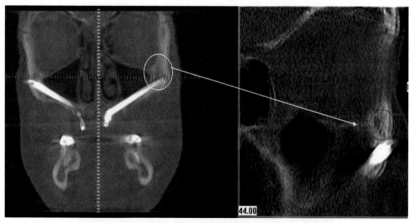

Fig. 55. CBCT examination of the patient's radiographs for placement of a second zygoma implant in the left zygomatic bone.

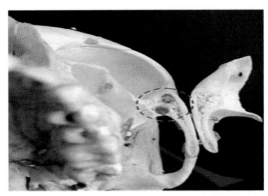

Fig. 56. Duel zygoma concepts; Stacking of the 2 implants one on top of the other.

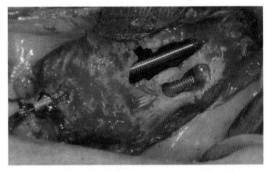

Fig. 57. Intraoperative view of the superior implant being placed.

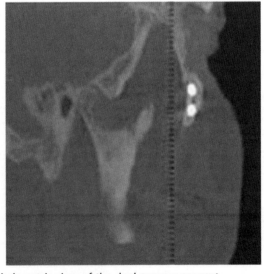

Fig. 58. CBCT, cephalometric view of the dual zygoma concept.

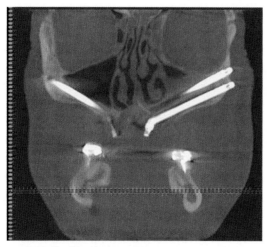

Fig. 59. Frontal view of the final implant positions.

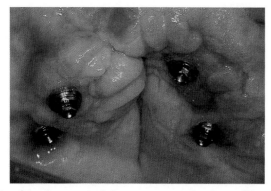

Fig. 60. Six months after placement of the new zygoma implant; all implants were asymptomatic and without mobility.

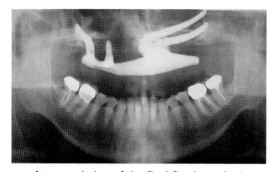

Fig. 61. Final panorex after completion of the final fixed prosthesis.

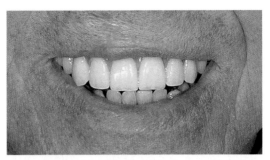

Fig. 62. Excellent aesthetics after fabrication of the final prosthesis.

DISCUSSION

Reported complications with the zygomatic implant include transient neurosensory disturbances, difficulty with speech, and sinus infections. Implant failures have also been reported.[14,15,19] Although the use of the zygomatic implant has been shown to be predictable with minimal postoperative complications, discussion of complications related to this procedure is warranted.

Neurosensory Disturbance

Neurosensory disturbance of the zygomaticofacial nerve has been reported due to encountering of this nerve during soft tissue reflection over the lateral aspect of the zygoma. A transient paresthesia was experienced in the 4 patients in this study[23] with resolution within the first 7 weeks postoperatively.

Difficulty with Speech

The resorption pattern of the posterior maxilla is toward the palate. The zygoma implant is generally placed in intimate contact with the lingual plate. In some cases, the prominence of the implant platform may be identifiable by the patients' tongue. However, adaptation to the lingual contour is usually well tolerated with minimal disruption of speech.[24]

Sinus Infections

Occurrences of maxillary sinus infection in patients who have undergone zygoma implant placement have been reported in the literature. Aparicio[15] reported delayed acute sinusitis at 14, 23, and 27 months after surgery. These infections resolved following oral antibiotics without further complications.

Most of the sinus infections reported were unilateral (**Fig. 63**) despite the presence of bilateral zygomatic implants. Therefore, the idea that the zygoma implant may, as a foreign body, be responsible for these infections seems unlikely.

Peterson[25] reported on foreign bodies in the maxillary sinus by reviewing patients 1 year after the placement of zygomatic implants. By introducing an endoscope used for rhinoscopy and sinoscopy through the lateral wall of the maxillary sinus (**Fig. 64**), he examined the state of the maxillary sinus, its associated membrane, and the portion of the zygoma implant traveling through the sinus. A 1-year follow-up of 14 subjects (**Fig. 65**) determined no signs of infection or inflammation in the mucosa around the fixtures. Therefore, the presence of unilateral infection in lieu of the presence of bilateral zygomatic implants suggests consideration of other causes than the implant itself.

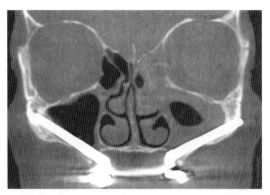

Fig. 63. Unilateral maxillary sinus infection after placement of zygoma implants.

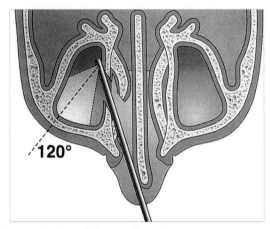

Fig. 64. Endoscopic examination of the maxillary sinus.

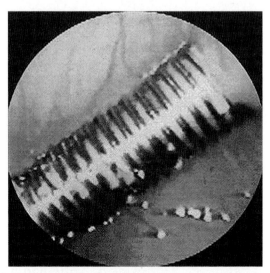

Fig. 65. Endoscopic view of the zygoma implant within the maxillary sinus without adverse reaction.

In the experience of this author, sinus infections are *late* infections, 12 to 24 months after the placement, and infections are generally unilateral. Most patients report having had a significant upper-respiratory infection that was followed by sinus congestion and pain. Symptoms include slight pressure over the anterior maxillary wall and occasional discharge from the nose. Oral antibiotics are initially prescribed. Once patients are refractory to 2 courses of oral antibiotics, an investigation into possible abnormal function of the meatus via 3-dimentional radiographic examination should be done.

The maxillary ostium is located in the superior aspect of the medial maxillary wall (**Fig. 66**). In order for the sinus to drain, a patent osteomeatal complex is necessary.

In cases where unilateral blockage occurs that is refractory to oral antibiotics, it is likely that drainage through the ostium is blocked secondary to inflammation. A functional endoscopic sinus surgery (FESS) is recommended.

Fig. 67 demonstrates the normal anatomy surrounding the maxillary ostium. The clinical photograph taken through a rigid endoscope also demonstrates the limited space between the nasal septum to the right and the lateral nasal wall (medial maxillary wall) to the left. A FESS procedure enlarges the maxillary ostium and allows drainage by removing the uncinate process, removing the middle turbinate, and unroofing of the ethmoidal air cells.

The postoperative figure and clinical photograph of a patient who has undergone the FESS procedure clearly shows the patency established after performing this procedure (**Fig. 68**).

Fig. 69 also demonstrates clear maxillary sinuses after having the FESS procedure performed with resultant drainage of the infection from the effected sinus.

In the experience of this author, 5 patients have been treated as previously described and all have completely recovered. All of these patients had bilateral zygoma implants placed but presented with unilateral, late infection, 12 to 60 months,

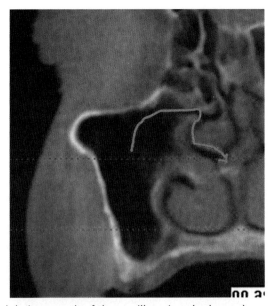

Fig. 66. Functional drainage path of the maxillary sinus (*red arrow*).

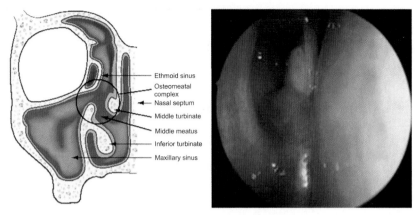

Fig. 67. Clinical view of the right naris before the FESS procedure.

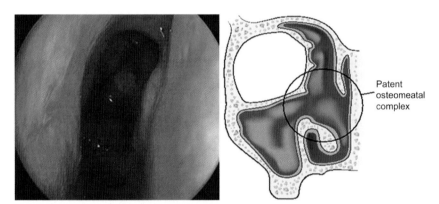

Fig. 68. Clinical view of the right naris after the FESS procedure.

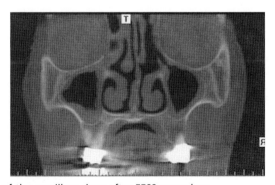

Fig. 69. Clearing of the maxillary sinus after FESS procedure.

after implant surgery with an immediate history of having recovered from an upper-respiratory infection. Therefore, referral of patients to an otolaryngologist for evaluation and treatment to establish a patent path for the drainage of the maxillary sinus is recommended.

SUMMARY

The management of the posterior maxilla with implant placement, including zygomatic implants, can be planned using the zones of available bone concept as a guideline. The use of anterior-tilted or posterior-tilted implants allows for establishing posterior implant support for a fixed prosthesis. The use of 2 premaxillary implants in conjunction with 2 posterior-tilted implants accomplishes this objective in a predictable manner. However, any of the implants may fail, interfering with the ability to continue use of the prosthesis. Presented here is the expanded use of the zygoma implant as a "rescue implant". The removal of a failed implant is immediately replaced with a zygoma implant to reestablish support needed for continuation of the prosthesis. In cases of rare, usually unilateral sinus infection associated with zygomatic implants, the physiologic drainage of the osteomeatal complex must evaluated and be attended to, including the possible need for a FESS procedure.

REFERENCES

1. Wood M, Vermilyea SG. A review of selected dental literature on evidence-based treatment planning for dental implants: report of the Committee on Research in Fixed Prosthodontics of the Academy of Fixed Prosthodontics. J Prosthet Dent 2004;92:447–62.
2. Breine U, Branemark PI. Reconstruction of alveolar jaw bone. An experimental and clinical study of immediate and performed autologous bone grafts in combination with osseointegrated implants. Scand J Plast Reconstr Surg 1980;14: 23–48.
3. Isaksson S, Ekfeld A, Alberius P, et al. Early results from reconstruction of severely atrophic (class VI) maxillas by immediate endosseous implants in conjunction with bone grafting and Lefort I osteotomy. J Oral Maxillofac Surg 1993;22:144–8.
4. Adell R, lekholm U, Grondal K, et al. Reconstruction of severely resorbed edentulous maxillae using osseointegrated fixtures in immediate autogenous grafts. Int J Oral Maxillofac Implants 1990;5:233–46.
5. Isaksson S, Alberius P. Maxillary alveolar ridge augmentation with only bone grafts and immediate endosseous implants. J Craniomaxillofac Surg 1992;20: 2–7.
6. Jensen OT, Shulman LB, Block MS, et al. Report of the sinus consensus conference of 1996. Int J Oral Maxillofac Implants 1998;13(Suppl):11–32.
7. Fortin Y, Sullivan RM, Rangert BR. The Marius implant bridge: surgical and prosthetic rehabilitation for the completely edentulous upper jaw with moderate to severe resorption: a 5-year retrospective clinical study. Clin Implant Dent Relat Res 2002;4:69–77.
8. Krekmanov L, Kahn M, Rangert B, et al. Tilting of posterior mandibular and maxillary implants for improved prosthesis support. Int J Oral Maxillofac Implants 2000;15:405–14.
9. Aparicio C, Perales P, Rangert B. Tilted implants as an alternative to maxillary sinus grafting: a clinical, radiologic, and periotest study. Clin Implant Dent Relat Res 2001;1:39–49.

10. Stevenson AR, Austin BW. Zygomatic fixtures- the Sydney experience. Ann R Australas Coll Dent Surg 2000;15:337.
11. Higuchi KW. The zygomatic fixture: an alternative approach for implant anchorage in the posterior maxilla. Ann R Australas Coll Dent Surg 2000;15: 28–33.
12. Bedrossian E, Stumpel LJ. The zygomatic implant; preliminary data on treatment of severely resorbed maxillae. A clinical report. Int J Oral Maxillofac Implants 2002;17:861–5.
13. Malevez C, Abarca M, Durdu F, et al. Clinical outcome of 103 consecutive zygomatic implants: a 6–48 month follow-up study. Clin Oral Implants Res 2004;115: 18–22.
14. Branemark PI, Grondal K, Ohrnell LO, et al. Zygoma fixture in the management of advanced atrophy of the maxilla: technique and long-term results. Scand J Plast Reconstr Surg Hand Surg 2004;38:70–85.
15. Aparicio C, Ouazzani W, Garcia R, et al. A prospective clinical study on titanium implants in the zygomatic arch for prosthetic rehabilitation of the atrophic maxilla a follow-up of 6 months to 5 years. Clin Implant Dent Relat Res 2006;8:114–22.
16. Bedrossian E, Rangert B, Stumpel L, et al. Immediate function with the zygomatic implant- a graftless solution for the patient with mild to advanced atrophy of the maxilla. Int J Oral Maxillofac Implants 2006;21(6):937–42.
17. Chow J, Hui E, Lee P, et al. Zygomatic implants-protocol for immediate loading: a preliminary report. J Oral Maxillofac Surg 2006;64:804–11.
18. Davo R, Malevez C, Rojas J. Immediate function in the atrophic maxilla using zygomatic implants: a preliminary study. J Prosthet Dent 2007;97:S44–51.
19. Bedrossian E. Rehabilitation of the edentulous maxilla with the zygoma concept: a 7 year prospective study. Int J Oral Maxillofac Implants 2010;25:1213–21.
20. Nkenke E, Hahn M, Lell M, et al. Anatomic site evaluation of the zygomatic bone for dental implant placement. Clin Oral Implants Res 2003;14:72–9.
21. Bedrossian E, Stumpel L. Immediate stabilization at phase II of zygomaticus fixtures; a simplified technique. J Prosthet Dent 2001;86(1):10–4.
22. Zhao Y, Skalak R, Branemark PI. Analysis of a dental prosthesis supported by zygomatic fixtures. Gothenberg (Sweden): The Insitue for Applied Biotechnology.
23. Reichert TE, Kunkel M, Wahlmann U, et al. [The zygomatic implant indications and first clinical experiences]. Zeitschrift fur Zahnärztliche Implantologie 1999; 15:65–70 [in German].
24. Bothur S, Garsten M. Initial speech problems in patients treated with multiple zygomatic implants. Int J Oral Maxillofac Implants 2010;5:379–84.
25. Petruson B. Sinoscopy in patients with titanium implants in the nose and sinuses. Scand J Plast Reconstr Surg Hand Surg 2004;38:86–93.

Maxillary All-On-Four Therapy Using Angled Implants: A 16-Month Clinical Study of 1110 Implants in 276 Jaws

Stuart Graves, DDS, MS[a],*, Brian A. Mahler, DDS[b], Ben Javid, DDS[c],
Debora Armellini, DDS, MD[d], Ole T. Jensen, DDS, MS[e,f]

KEYWORDS

- Maxillary implants • All-on-Four implant protocol
- Tilted implants • Edentulous maxilla
- Pterygomaxillary implants • Zygomatic implants

The maxilla is a challenging area for dental implant restoration. Encroachment of anatomic structures such as the sinus and nasal floor make vertical placement difficult. Implants placed at an angle may be used to avoid these anatomic structures or eliminate the need for a bone grafting procedure. The question occasionally arises about the possible detrimental effects of placing implants at an angle. It should be noted that because of bone resorption numerous implants, especially in the maxillary anterior, have been placed at significant angles for many years. Anecdotally these tilted implants seem to work, but what evidence is available in the literature with regard to the efficacy of implants placed at an angle?

This article was previously published in the May 2011 issue of *Oral and Maxillofacial Surgery Clinics of North America*.

[a] Northern Virginia Oral Maxillofacial & Implant Surgery, Burke Professional Center, 5206 Lyngate Court, Burke, VA 22015, USA

[b] Private Practice, 10550 Warwick Avenue, Fairfax, VA 22030, USA

[c] ClearChoice Dental Implant Center–Washington Metro, 11200 Rockville Pike, Suite 115, Bethesda, MD 20852, USA

[d] ClearChoice Dental Implant Center–Washington Metro, 8219 Leesburg Pike, Suite 100, Vienna, VA 22182, USA

[e] Implant Dentistry Associates of Colorado, 8200 East Belleview Avenue, Suite 520E, Greenwood Village, CO 80111, USA

[f] Department of Oral and Maxillofacial Surgery, Hebrew University School of Dental Medicine, POB 12272, Jerusalem, 91120, Israel

* Corresponding author.

E-mail address: stuart.graves@clearchoice.com

A literature search was conducted regarding the placement of off axis implants. It has been concluded by some using Finite Element Analysis, mathematical models,[1–11] and mechanical testing[12] that off-axis loading will produce more stress on the implant and implant/bone interface, although the 2 articles that speculated on the possible results of these forces believed the forces would be within the physiologic range for the most part. In other studies[13–17] Finite Element Analysis concluded that, under many common clinical situations, no stress differences were apparent between tilted and nontilted implants. Two animal studies[18,19] showed no apparent long-term differences in hard or soft tissue results around nonaxial implants, although one[19] showed short-term differences in the healing mechanisms.

Although mathematical models, mechanical testing, and animal studies can provide useful information, long-term human clinical results are required to ensure a procedure is effective. There have been numerous studies and articles published regarding tilted implants in humans.

Implants placed into the pterygomaxillary regions were some of the first implants intentionally tilted. Such implants have been used for more than 20 years. Pterygomaxillary implants often allow for the placement of implants in the posterior maxilla without the use of sinus augmentation procedures or other types of bone grafts. This method decreases the cost of implant treatment and saves time, eliminating the need for cantilevers in many cases. Balshi and colleagues[20] found the survival rate of these implants to be comparable to previous studies for implants placed in the maxillary arch. A subsequently published study[21] by the same investigators using surface-roughened implants in the pterygomaxillary region showed excellent clinical results. Valerón and Valerón[22] followed pterygomaxillary implants for a minimum of 5 years and up to 10 years. These investigators lost only 2 of 152 implants after functional loading, and concluded that despite the necessity for inclination, these implants easily supported functional load. It should be noted that these implants are often placed into the worst quality bone and under the highest forces possible. The majority of the implants in most studies were 4.0 mm or less in diameter. All articles on these off-axis implants in the pterygomaxillary region appear to endorse their use.

Another implant that is intentionally placed at an angle is the zygomatic implant. These implants have also been used for more than 15 years. Three studies concluded that these implants are a predictable alternative to extensive bone grafting.[23–25] Two other articles found acceptable results but advocated further studies.[26,27] None of these articles referenced concern regarding adverse outcomes due to the angulations of these implants.

Implants placed off-axis usually require angle-corrected abutments. Eger and colleagues[28] concluded that implants placed at unfavorable angles may be restored with angled abutments without compromise of function or esthetics. Sethi and colleagues[29,30] published 2 articles following 3100 angle-corrected restorations over 10 years, concluding that good esthetic and functional results can be achieved. Koutouzis and Wennström[31] compared bone levels of fixed partial dentures restored on implants at 5 years that used both axial and nonaxial placed implants, and concluded that implant inclination had no effect on peri-implant bone loss.

Articles have been published using intentionally tilted implants in other locations. Krekmanov and colleagues[32] followed cases for up to 5 years that involved the tilting of implants distally anterior to both the sinus and the mental foramen, and concluded that this method of treatment for edentulous arches represents an alternative or complementary technique to others mentioned in the literature. The investigators stated that this technique leads to an improved position of support, and allows for placement of longer implants and/or improved anchorage in dense bone. Biomechanical measurements showed that the tilting does not have a negative effect on the load distribution when it is a part of prosthesis support. The advantages are further extension of the prosthesis in a posterior direction, possible use of longer posterior implants, and improved bone anchorage. Krekmanov and colleagues concluded that the technique is relatively easy to perform in any outpatient setting by a surgeon who is not familiar with bone grafting of the maxillary sinus. Furthermore, it eliminates the need for such advanced techniques for some patients.

Maló and colleagues[33] used implants in the maxilla and mandible in a similar manner to Krekmanov except that most implants were immediately restored. At 1 year Maló and colleagues concluded that this treatment modality was highly successful. Four additional studies[34–38] used a similar technique, immediately restoring the maxilla and/or mandible with full-arch fixed prostheses. All 3 studies found similar bone levels, and all 3 concluded that tilted implants may be a viable treatment modality.

Rosén and Gynther[39] followed implants in the maxilla for 8 to 12 years that were tilted to avoid grafting procedures, concluding that this was a successful alternative procedure to the more resource-demanding techniques involving bone grafting. Calandriello and Tomatis[40] showed similar finding in a 1-year follow-up study. Krennmair and colleagues[41] studied 62 patients with overdentures and analyzed the various angles of the implants placed for optimal restoration. It was concluded that sagittal inclination should be attributed more importance than axial loading of implants. Aparicio and colleagues[42] followed fixed implant bridges supported by both axial and tilted implants for 21 to 87 months after insertion. Fortin and colleagues[43,44] followed intentionally placed tilted implants using an image-guided system in the atrophic maxilla over 4 years. Both of these groups concluded that the use of tilted implants is an effective and safe alternative to maxillary sinus floor augmentation procedures.

METHODS

The All-on-Four protocol as set forth by Maló and colleagues[33] for immediately rehabilitating the edentulous maxilla was used for fully edentulous patients as well as being applied to partially dentate patients who preferred a fixed alternative to an interim removable denture during implant healing. This series spans a homologous group treated by the same surgical-prosthetic team over the course of 16 months using extractions when indicated, simultaneous implant placement, and immediate loading (within 3–6 hours post surgery) with a fixed acrylic hybrid prosthesis. A total of 1110 implants were placed in 276 maxillas. Nine maxillas were not loaded on the day of surgery, due to insufficient torque values for immediate loading. Forty-five definitive prostheses have been delivered to date. All surgeries were completed under intravenous anesthesia.

PATIENT SELECTION AND PREOPERATIVE PROCEDURE

All patients underwent a comprehensive prosthetic examination, presurgical consultation with necessary medical consultations, and an anesthesia evaluation. Only American Society of Anesthesiologists grades I and II were treated. Patients were excluded if they demonstrated poorly controlled diabetes mellitus, active neoplastic disease, and history of bisphosphonate use with a fasting C-terminal telopeptide level below 150 pg/mL. Presurgical planning included cone-beam computed tomography, periapical radiographs where indicated, impressions, and records necessary for fabrication of the interim prosthesis before surgery.

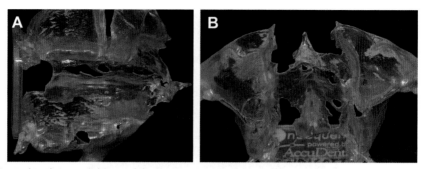

Fig. 5. (A, B) Stereolithic models demonstrate severe atrophy.

protocol of Stella and Warner,[45] a lateral slot technique was used in both right and left maxillary sinuses and two 42.5-mm TiUnite implants (Nobel Biocare) placed. Cover screws were placed on all implants, and the area was sutured with 3-0 chromic in a running suture. Hemostasis was good and the patient's existing upper denture was relined.

The patient's mandible was treated in a conventional fashion for an All-on-Four prosthesis. Parallel crestal incisions approximately 3 mm apart were used to expose the superior half of the mandible with sharp bisection. The mental foramina were exposed, the bone tabled to a flat surface, and 4 active implants placed. The bicuspid area was 15 mm and the lateral incisor area was 13 mm. All lower implants achieved torque values of approximately 50 Ncm. The incisions were closed with interrupted 3-0 chromic. Angled abutments were placed, 30° posteriorly and 17° anteriorly.

Prosthetic Procedure

Following surgery, an interim maxillary denture was soft-lined and delivered. Next, abutment level impression copings were placed on the mandibular implants and linked using pattern resin and wire. An impression was made using an open-tray technique. While the impression was poured, temporary cylinders were attached to the implants and the previously fabricated lower interim prosthesis was related to the cylinders using acrylic resin. Care was taken to maintain the horizontal plane orientation and maintain the preestablished vertical dimension of occlusion by using a closed-mouth technique. A laboratory reline procedure was completed for the lower prosthesis prior to same-day delivery. At interim prosthesis delivery prosthetic screws

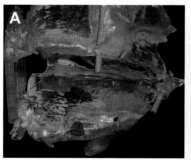
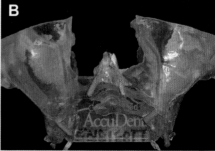

Fig. 6. (A, B) Implants were placed in the models in a "mock surgery."

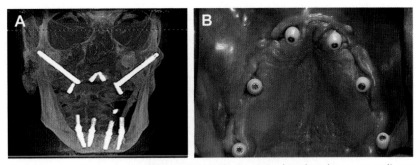

Fig. 7. (*A*) Zygomatic, vomer, and pterygoid implants were placed as shown on radiograph. (*B*) The implants were uncovered after 6 months.

were torqued to 15 Ncm and access holes were sealed with gingival retraction cord and "Fermit." Group function was verified and the patient was advised to maintain a soft diet during the integration period.

Six months later, second-stage uncovering of the maxillary implants was performed in the usual fashion (see **Fig. 7**). The appropriate angled abutments were placed so that the screw access holes did not reach the facies of any teeth. Approximately 1 month later, impressions were made for both upper and lower definitive prostheses. The completed full-arch prostheses were supported by a milled titanium framework with cantilevers to allow for maximum posterior occlusion. After appointments verifying the accuracy of the bar and the occlusion, final restorations were delivered 3 months later (**Figs. 8 and 9**).

CASE 2

A 42-year old woman had worn dentures for less than 2 years following what she described as 7 years of aggressive periodontal treatment and subsequent extractions (**Figs. 10 and 11**). She reported wearing a removable denture that had detrimental effects on both her social as well as psychological well-being. Upper and lower implants were planned along with extraction of remaining failing lower teeth (**Figs. 12 and 13**).

Surgical Procedure

The patient was premedicated with clindamycin, 600 mg, 1 hour before surgery. She was also given 0.1% chlorhexidine rinse. She was sedated intravenously using a local

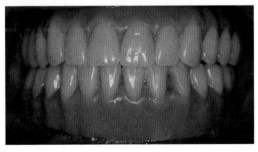

Fig. 8. Final restoration.

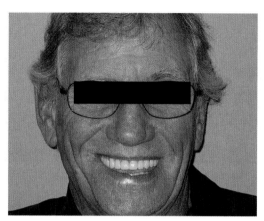

Fig. 9. Final restoration.

anesthetic of septocaine and maracaine that were administered in both the maxilla and mandible. In the edentulous maxilla, it was decided to remove 4 mm of vertical height of bone. With this in mind, a buccal incision was made 3 mm to the outside of the crest. A similar incision, parallel to this, was made on the lingual. These incisions were joined to the tuberosity with sharp dissection. The buccal and lingual tissues were elevated, exposing the anterior floor of the nose, the zygomatic buttress, and the pterygoid fissure (**Figs. 14–17**). Using a reciprocating saw, the maxillary bone was sectioned to a uniformed height on both sides of the maxilla. A Fox Plane was used to assess the horizontal accuracy of the cut. The bone was then smoothed using a reciprocal file. The architecture of the surface was identified with transillumination. The anterior wall of the sinus was then outlined with a permanent marker.

NobelActive implants were placed just anterior to the floor of the sinus at a 30° angle to the occlusal plane. These implants were used according to the protocol as dictated by Nobel for the 4.3-mm implant. Two 4.3×18-mm implants were placed bilaterally and torqued to a force of 50 Ncm. Using a prefabricated surgical guide, locations for the anterior were determined. Both of these were between the canine and lateral incisor area. These implants were also placed at a 17° angle to the occlusal plane.

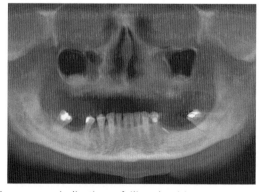

Fig. 10. Preoperative panorex indicating a failing dentition.

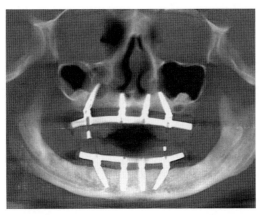

Fig. 11. Postoperative panorex with All-on-Four implants in place.

The apical portion of the implant engaged the floor of the nose. All of the implants were counter-sunk using the dedicated bone mill. Multi-unit abutments were then torqued into place on all of the implants, consisting of 17° in the anterior and the 30° in the posterior. Healing caps were then placed on the abutments and the soft tissue was closed with interrupted 3-0 chromic sutures.

Attention was then turned to the mandible, where all the remaining teeth were extracted and 4 implants placed in a very similar protocol to the upper arch. Slightly

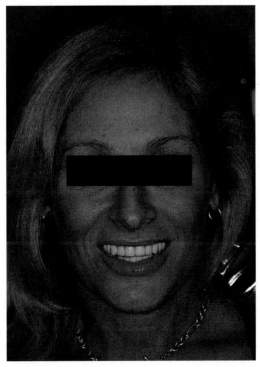

Fig. 12. Final restoration.

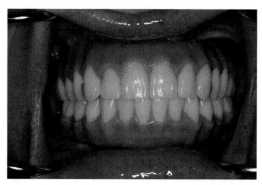

Fig. 13. Final restoration.

more bone (6 mm) was tabled on the lower jaw. All of the implants were torqued to 50 Ncm. Abutments were then placed as described for the maxillary arch.

Prosthetic Procedure

Following surgery, abutment level impression copings were placed on the maxillary implants. Seating of the impression copings was verified by periapical radiographs (**Fig. 18**). Copings were then linked using pattern resin and wire. An impression was made using an open-tray technique. While the impression was poured, temporary cylinders were attached to the implants and the previously fabricated upper and lower interim prostheses were related to the cylinders using acrylic resin. Care was taken to maintain the horizontal plane orientation and maintain the preestablished vertical dimension of occlusion by using a closed-mouth technique. A laboratory reline procedure was completed for both prostheses prior to same-day delivery. At delivery prosthetic screws were torqued to 15 Ncm, and access holes were sealed with gingival retraction cord and Fermit. Anterior occlusion and posterior disclusion were verified, and the patient was advised to maintain a soft diet during the integration period.

Final impressions for the definitive maxillary and mandibular fixed-hybrid prostheses were performed 6 months after surgery (**Fig. 19**). The completed full-arch prostheses were supported by milled titanium frameworks with cantilevers to allow for maximum posterior occlusion.

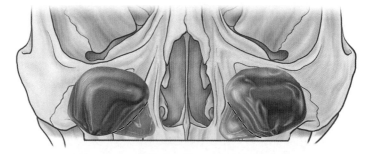

Fig. 14. When there is minimal paranasal bone available for implant placement and sinus anatomy is prominent, sometimes even deflecting anterior of the canine eminence, transsinus implants can be considered.

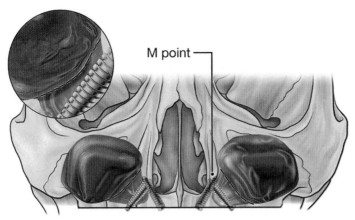

Fig. 15. Following sinus membrane elevation, the distal implant is placed transsinus to engage "M" point.

At delivery, occlusion was verified and prosthetic screws were torqued to 15 Ncm. Access holes were sealed with gingival retraction cord and Fermit. At 3 months after delivery, after verifying screws were torqued to 15 Ncm, access holes were sealed with retraction cord and composite.

RESULTS

From July 2009 to November 2010, 276 patients received implant treatment involving angled implants in the maxilla. Two hundred and sixty-seven patients received fixed interim prostheses on the day of surgery. Forty-five patients received final prostheses. The patient population included dentate as well as edentulous individuals. Age, smoking history, or systemic disease controlled by medication was not a criterion for discussion. Failure is defined as inability to withstand 35 Ncm of torque 6 months postoperatively. In all, 1110 implants were placed, with 28 failures and a success rate of 97.48%.

Anteroposterior spread was measured in all cases. Distance was measured between a line through the center of the frontmost implants and a line through the posterior implants. The two sides were averaged. The average distance was 15.9 mm. Of note, on mandibular arches in the same patient population this measurement was less, at 15.25 mm.

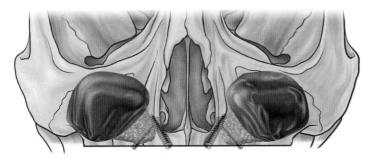

Fig. 16. The exposed implant, including the sinus floor, is then bone grafted using BMP-2.

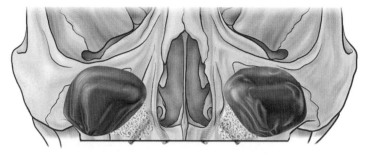

Fig. 17. Late term healing consolidates the graft after 4 months.

A large majority of the published data has substantiated that angled implants are a valid and indeed beneficial treatment modality for the maxilla. This type of implant treatment has become more commonplace over time with an increasing number of advocates in the literature. Numerous possible benefits of the tilted placement of implants are found in the literature, and these include:

1. Elimination of bone grafting procedures resulting in:
   Shorter total treatment time
   Less patient morbidity
   Decreased cost
   Possible immediate restoration not available in conjunction with most bone grafting procedures
2. Increase in anterior-posterior spread, resulting in a more stable prosthesis

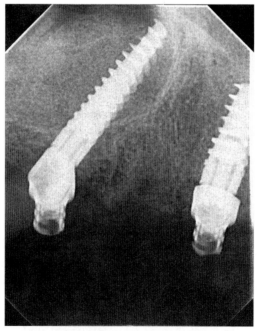

Fig. 18. A periapical radiograph showing a posterior All-on-Four implant passing transsinus to engage paranasal bone at "M" point.

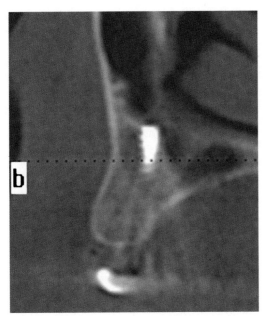

Fig. 19. After 6 months of healing, the implant appears well integrated into consolidated sinus graft, the tip of the implant engaging into the lateral nasal wall.

3. Elimination or shortening of cantilevers
4. Avoidance of various anatomic structures
5. Fewer implants to support the prosthesis.

The placement of angled implants has numerous benefits to patients. The placement of these implants into the patient's available bone is usually easier for the surgical dentist than additional grafting procedures.

One possible disadvantage of the tilted placement of conventional dental implants is that they usually become more difficult to restore, which requires angle-correcting abutments. These abutments are available in different angles from most implant manufacturers. Care must be taken to create enough vertical space for the intermediate abutment.

REFERENCES

1. Sütpideler M, Eckert SE, Zobitz M, et al. Finite element analysis of effect of prosthesis height, angle of force application, and implant offset on supporting bone. Int J Oral Maxillofac Implants 2004;19(6):819–25.
2. Saab XE, Griggs JA, Powers JM, et al. Effect of abutment angulation on the strain on the bone around an implant in the anterior maxilla: a finite element study. J Prosthet Dent 2007;97(2):85–92.
3. Cehreli MC, Iplikçioğlu H, Bilir OG. The influence of the location of load transfer on strains around implants supporting four unit cement-retained fixed prostheses: in vitro evaluation of axial versus non-axial loading. J Oral Rehabil 2002;29(4):394–400.
4. Brosh T, Pilo R, Sudai D. The influence of abutment angulation on strains and stresses along the implant/bone interface: comparison between 2 experimental techniques. J Prosthet Dent 1998;79:328–34.

5. Clelland NL, Lee JK, Bimbenet OC, et al. A three-dimensional finite element stress analysis of angled abutments for an implant placed in the anterior maxilla. J Prosthodont 1995;4:95–100.

6. Cehreli MC, Iplikçioğlu H. In vitro strain analysis and off-axial loading on implant supported fixed partial dentures. Implant Dent 2002;11(3):286–92.

7. O'Mahony A, Bowles Q, Woolsey G, et al. Stress distribution in the single-unit osseointegrated dental implant: finite element analyses of axial and off-axial loading. Implant Dent 2000;9(3):207–18.

8. Hsu ML, Chen FC, Kao HC, et al. Influence of off-axis loading of an anterior maxillary implant: a 3-dimensional finite element analysis. Int J Oral Maxillofac Implants 2007;22(2):301–9.

9. Zampelis A, Rangert B, Heijl L. Tilting of splinted implants for improved prosthodontic support: a two-dimensional finite element analysis. J Prosthet Dent 2007; 97(Suppl 6):S35–43.

10. Lin CL, Wang JC, Ramp LC, et al. Biomechanical response of implant systems placed in the maxillary posterior region under various conditions of angulation, bone density, and loading. Int J Oral Maxillofac Implants 2008;23(1):57–64.

11. Kao HC, Gung YW, Chung TF, et al. The influence of abutment angulation on micromotion level for immediately loaded dental implants: a 3-D finite element analysis. Int J Oral Maxillofac Implants 2008;23(4):623–30.

12. Clelland NL, Gilat A, McGlumphy EA, et al. A photoelastic and strain gauge analysis of angled abutments for an implant system. Int J Oral Maxillofac Implants 1993;8(5):541–8.

13. Cruz M, Wassall T, Toledo EM, et al. Finite element stress analysis of dental prostheses supported by straight and angled implants. Int J Oral Maxillofac Implants 2009;24(3):391–403.

14. Bellini CM, Romeo D, Galbusera F, et al. A finite element analysis of tilted versus non-tilted implant configurations in the edentulous maxilla. Int J Prosthodont 2009;22(2):155–7.

15. Las Casas EB, Ferreira PC, Cimini CA Jr, et al. Comparative 3D finite element stress analysis of straight and angled wedge-shaped implant designs. Int J Oral Maxillofac Implants 2008;23(2):215–25.

16. Markarian RA, Ueda C, Sendyk CL, et al. Stress distribution after installation of fixed frameworks with marginal gaps over angled and parallel implants: a photoelastic analysis. J Prosthodont 2007;16(2):117–22.

17. Bellini CM, Romeo D, Galbusera F, et al. Comparison of tilted versus nontilted implant-supported prosthetic designs for the restoration of the edentulous mandible: a biomechanical study. Int J Oral Maxillofac Implants 2009;24(3):511–7.

18. Celletti R, Pameijer CH, Bracchetti G, et al. Histologic evaluation of osseointegrated implants restored in nonaxial functional occlusion with preangled abutments. Int J Periodontics Restorative Dent 1995;15(6):562–73.

19. Barbier L, Schepers E. Adaptive bone remodeling around oral implants under axial and nonaxial loading conditions in the dog mandible. Int J Oral Maxillofac Implants 1997;12(2):215–23.

20. Balshi SF, Wolfinger GJ, Balshi TJ. Analysis of 356 pterygomaxillary implants in edentulous arches for fixed prosthesis anchorage. Int J Oral Maxillofac Implants 1999;14(3):398–406.

21. Balshi SF, Wolfinger GJ, Balshi TJ. Analysis of 164 titanium oxide-surface implants in completely edentulous arches for fixed prosthesis anchorage using the pterygomaxillary region. Int J Oral Maxillofac Implants 2005;20(6):946–52.

22. Valerón JF, Valerón PF. Long-term results in placement of screw-type implants in the pterygomaxillary-pyramidal region. Int J Oral Maxillofac Implants 2007;22(2): 195–200.
23. Ahlgren F, Størksen K, Tornes K. A study of 25 zygomatic dental implants with 11 to 49 months' follow-up after loading. Int J Oral Maxillofac Implants 2006;21(3): 421–5.
24. Aparicio C, Ouazzani W, Garcia R, et al. A prospective clinical study on titanium implants in the zygomatic arch for prosthetic rehabilitation of the atrophic edentulous maxilla with a follow-up of 6 months to 5 years. Clin Implant Dent Relat Res 2006;8(3):114–22.
25. Bedrossian E, Rangert B, Stumpel L, et al. Immediate function with the zygomatic implant: a graftless solution for the patient with mild to advanced atrophy of the maxilla. Int J Oral Maxillofac Implants 2006;21(6):937–42.
26. Becktor JP, Isaksson S, Abrahamsson P, et al. Evaluation of 31 zygomatic implants and 74 regular dental implants used in 16 patients for prosthetic reconstruction of the atrophic maxilla with cross-arch fixed bridges. Clin Implant Dent Relat Res 2005;7(3):159–65.
27. Farzad P, Andersson L, Gunnarsson S, et al. Rehabilitation of severely resorbed maxillae with zygomatic implants: an evaluation of implant stability, tissue conditions, and patients' opinion before and after treatment. Int J Oral Maxillofac Implants 2006;21(3):399–404.
28. Eger DE, Gunsolley JC, Feldman S. Comparison of angled and standard abutments and their effect on clinical outcomes: a preliminary report. Int J Oral Maxillofac Implants 2000;15(6):819–23.
29. Sethi A, Kaus T, Sochor P. The use of angulated abutments in implant dentistry: five-year clinical results of an ongoing prospective study. Int J Oral Maxillofac Implants 2000;15(6):801–10.
30. Sethi A, Kaus T, Sochor P, et al. Evolution of the concept of angulated abutments in implant dentistry: 14-year clinical data. Implant Dent 2002;11(1):41–51.
31. Koutouzis T, Wennström JL. Bone level changes at axial- and non-axial-positioned implants supporting fixed partial dentures. A 5-year retrospective longitudinal study. Clin Oral Implants Res 2007;18(5):585–90.
32. Krekmanov L, Kahn M, Rangert B, et al. Tilting of posterior mandibular and maxillary implants for improved prosthesis support. Int J Oral Maxillofac Implants 2000;15(3):405–14.
33. Maló P, Nobre Mde A, Petersson U, et al. A pilot study of complete edentulous rehabilitation with immediate function using a new implant design: case series. Clin Implant Dent Relat Res 2006;8(4):223–32.
34. Francetti L, Agliardi E, Testori T, et al. Immediate rehabilitation of the mandible with fixed full prosthesis supported by axial and tilted implants: interim results of a single cohort prospective study. Clin Implant Dent Relat Res 2008;10(4): 255–63.
35. Testori T, Del Fabbro M, Capelli M, et al. Immediate occlusal loading and tilted implants for the rehabilitation of the atrophic edentulous maxilla: 1-year interim results of a multicenter prospective study. Clin Oral Implants Res 2008;19(3): 227–32.
36. Capelli M, Zuffettii F, Del Fabbro M, et al. Immediate rehabilitation of the completely edentulous jaw with fixed prostheses supported by either upright or tilted implants: a multicenter clinical study. Int J Oral Maxillofac Implants 2007; 22(4):639–44.

37. Agliardi EL, Francetti L, Romeo D, et al. Immediate loading in the fully edentulous maxilla without bone grafting: the V-II-V technique. Minerva Stomatol 2008;57(5): 251–63.

38. Agliardi EL, Francetti L, Romeo D, et al. Immediate rehabilitation of the edentulous maxilla: preliminary results of a single-cohort prospective study. Int J Oral Maxillofac Implants 2009;24(5):887–95.

39. Rosén A, Gynther G. Implant treatment without bone grafting in edentulous severely resorbed maxillas: a long-term follow-up study. J Oral Maxillofac Surg 2007;65(5):1010–6.

40. Calandriello R, Tomatis M. Simplified treatment of the atrophic posterior maxilla via immediate/early function and tilted implants: a prospective 1-year clinical study. Clin Implant Dent Relat Res 2005;7(Suppl 1):S1–12.

41. Krennmair G, Fürhauser R, Krainhöfner M, et al. Clinical outcome and prosthodontic compensation of tilted interforaminal implants for mandibular overdentures. Int J Oral Maxillofac Implants 2005;20(6):923–9.

42. Aparicio C, Perales P, Rangert B. Tilted implants as an alternative to maxillary sinus grafting: a clinical, radiologic, and periotest study. Clin Implant Dent Relat Res 2001;3(1):39–49.

43. Fortin T, Isidori M, Bouchet H. Placement of posterior maxillary implants in partially edentulous patients with severe bone deficiency using CAD/CAM guidance to avoid sinus grafting: a clinical report of procedure. Int J Oral Maxillofac Implants 2009;24(1):96–102.

44. Bevilacqua M, Tealdo T, Pera F, et al. Three-dimensional finite element analysis of load transmission using different implant inclinations and cantilever lengths. Int J Prosthodont 2008;21(6):539–42.

45. Stella JP, Warner MR. Sinus slot technique for simplification and improved orientation of Zygomaticus dental implants: a technical note. Int J Oral Maxillofac Implants 2000;15(6):889–93.

Mandibular All-On-Four Therapy Using Angled Implants: A Three-Year Clinical Study of 857 Implants in 219 Jaws

Caesar C. Butura, DDS[a],*, Daniel F. Galindo, DDS[a],
Ole T. Jensen, DDS, MS[b,c]

KEYWORDS

- All-on-Four procedure • Implants • Angled fixtures
- Full-arch restoration

The original Brånemark surgical-prosthetic protocol advocated the placement of four implant fixtures for the restoration of a resorbed mandible and six implant fixtures on mandibles that demonstrated minimal to moderate resorption.[1] Brånemark positioned the fixtures between the mental nerves, thus taking advantage of high cortical density.[2] This symphyseal position, however, also became a limiting factor with respect to the ability to extend the prosthesis posteriorly. Vertical implant placement required the prosthesis to have cantilever lengths of 10 to 20 mm to provide adequate function and aesthetic outcome. Biomechanical studies then demonstrated that regardless of the number of implants used, cantilever spans should not exceed 7 mm to provide optimal stability[3,4] as extended cantilevers demonstrate double the compressive forces on the distal-most implant.[5]

This article was previously published in the May 2011 issue of *Oral and Maxillofacial Surgery Clinics of North America*.
[a] ClearChoice Dental Implant Center, 20830 North Tatum Boulevard, Suite 150, Phoenix, AZ 85050, USA
[b] Implant Dentistry Associates of Colorado, 8200 East Belleview Avenue, Suite 520E, Greenwood Village, CO 80111, USA
[c] Department of Oral and Maxillofacial Surgery, Hebrew University School of Dental Medicine, POB 12272, Jerusalem 91120, Israel
* Corresponding author.
E-mail address: cbutura@clearchoice.com

Dent Clin N Am 55 (2011) 795–811
doi:10.1016/j.cden.2011.07.015
0011-8532/11/$ – see front matter © 2011 Elsevier Inc. All rights reserved.

Multiple surgical solutions arose out of the need to provide improved implant positions for the posterior mandible and decrease the length of the distal cantilever. Jensen and Nock[6] first described repositioning of the inferior alveolar nerve (IAN) for the placement of endosseous dental implants. Brånemark[7] and Jensen[8] also used IAN repositioning to facilitate placement of dental implants in the atrophic posterior mandible.[8] However, lateralizing the IAN to facilitate implant placement produced neurosensory disturbance, the recovery of which was not always certain.[9] Therefore, nerve lateralization was rarely done.

The simple solution of placement of angled implants appeared to solve this problem as it greatly reduced cantilever length while improving anterior-posterior (A-P) spread and thereby stability of the prosthesis. Krekmanov[10] was able to decrease the posterior cantilever length by simply tilting the distal-most implant. The angulation of the distal implant was also found to reduce tensile stress of the prosthesis.[11] Two-dimensional finite elemental analysis showed that the use of cantilevers resulted in higher stress at the marginal bone.[12] Reduction of the cantilever arm by the use of an apically tilted implant mitigated this stress pattern.[13]

The use of distal-angled implants for the support of fixed hybrid prostheses has now been reported as a viable alternative to grafting and nerve lateralization.[14–18] Further work by Krekmanov and Aparicio[19–21] showed that tilted implants did not exhibit advanced or extreme bone loss nor did they demonstrate significant bone stress when compared with cantilevers on vertically placed implants.

The next question is: Could tilted implants be immediately loaded? Initial work on immediately loading of nonangulated mandibular implants came from Schnitman and Wohrle, reporting a 10-year experience using Brånemark implants.[22] Since then, the concept of immediate-load full-arch splinted restorations in the edentulous mandible has been well documented by several authors with either four or six implant fixtures.[23–28] A comprehensive literature review on immediately loaded edentulous mandibles revealed a success rate between 98% and 100% over 1 to 3 years based on the use of four to eight implant fixtures.[29] The use of fewer implants was further studied by Malo and Rangert[30] with the application of the All-on-Four concept with the use of angulated fixtures. The technique employed four NobelBiocare Speedy TiUnite fixtures (Yorba Linda, CA, USA) with two anterior vertical and two posterior 30° angled fixtures. All implants underwent immediate loading with a splinted one-piece all acrylic full-arch restoration. A 1-year follow up demonstrated a prosthesis success rate of 100% and implant success rate of 96.7% to 98.2%, respectively. Khatami and colleagues[31] further validated the success of immediate loaded angulated implants in the edentulous mandible using the All-on-Four approach. The special category of the severely atrophic mandible was addressed by Jensen[32] who used a variation of the All-on-Four concept termed "V-4." This mandibular fracture-avoidance technique allowed for placement of implants in Cawood Class IV-V mandibles that had between 5 and 7 mm of basal bone available without bone grafting. All four implants were placed in a "V" formation, at 30° angles, all directed toward the symphysis where most bone mass remained.

The next question of importance was immediate loading in extraction sites: could this dependably be done? Placement of implants into immediate extraction sites had become a well accepted treatment option for single teeth but not for full-arch restorations, especially requiring multiple extractions.[33–35] The survival rate for immediately placed extraction site implants was reported from 91.8% to 99.5%, ranging from 1- to 11-years follow-up.[36,37] Villa and Rangert[38] reported on placement of dental implants into compromised extraction sites and loading with a provisional all-acrylic prosthesis within 3 days postoperatively. Implant success rate at 44 months was reported at 100% with marginal bone loss of 0.5 to 0.7 mm by the first year. Similar results were reported by Grunder[27] and, separately, by Cosci.[39] Using standard surgical and maintenance protocol, Malo and colleagues[40] reported a cumulative implant survival rate with immediate extraction, placement and loading of 100% after 1 year.[29] Also, marginal bone loss was comparable to previous studies. This was a very important finding. For the first time, full-arch immediate function in the dental extraction case appeared possible. However, there have been very few reports, with only a limited number of patients, since that time. For that reason, a retrospective study was done of 219 consecutive patients treated with angled implants using All-on-Four therapy in the mandible, the majority of which required dental extraction.

PATIENT SELECTION AND EVALUATION

A retrospective study of the All-on-Four protocol was done for both dentate and edentulous patients. The series spanned a diverse patient population treated by the same surgical-prosthetic team (Dental Implant Center, Phoenix, AZ, USA) over the course of 36 months. They performed dental extractions when indicated, simultaneous implant placement, and immediate loading (within 2–3 hours postsurgery) with a fixed acrylic hybrid prosthesis. A total of 857 implants were placed in 219 mandibles, of which 201 had more than three teeth present, 18 were fully edentulous, 7 had one to three teeth, 49 had four to six teeth, and 145 had over seven teeth. All surgeries were completed under monitored IV anesthesia.

The patient selection protocol consisted of a comprehensive prosthetic examination—presurgical consultation with necessary medical and anesthesia evaluations. Only ASA I and II patients were treated as defined by the American Society of Anesthesiologists. Patients were excluded if they demonstrated poorly controlled diabetes mellitus, active neoplastic disease, or a history of bisphosphonate use with a fasting collagen telepeptide (CTx) blood level below 150 pg/mL.

The prosthetic presurgical work-up included cone-beam CT scan (CBCT), and periapical and panoramic radiographs. Impressions of the maxilla and mandible were made, along with facebow transfer and interocclusal records.

Attention was given to the rest position of the lower lip and the relation of the lip to the remaining mandibular anterior dentition, if any, or the existing prosthesis. In order to provide a satisfactory aesthetic outcome, the junction between the prosthesis and the residual ridge needed to lie at least 10 mm apical to the inferior border of the lip. This ensured enough thickness of the prosthesis for structural integrity. The anticipated bone reduction was evaluated clinically and radiographically and noted on the surgical prescription.

RADIOGRAPHIC EVALUATION

Presurgical radiographic examination included CBCT to evaluate the anatomy of the mandible.[32,41] Height, width, cortical anatomy, and position of the IAN were evaluated using the CBCT software.[42,43] The mandible was examined with attention given to the IAN position and its course through the mandible. The anterior loop was identified to predict the need for nerve repositioning.

The CBCT studies were assessed for osseous pathology, arch shape, and bone volume. Mandibles that displayed a U-shape were differentiated from those which had more of a V-shaped anatomy. This finding helped determine implant positioning with regard to A-P spread. Patients with a flat U-shaped anatomy were informed of the possibility of IAN repositioning to avoid straight-line implant placement.

Edentulous atrophic mandibles often presented with tubular anatomy with absent or very poor medullary trabecular bone. Hounsfield unit values in the CBCT software were used to determine the porosity of the mandible. "Hollow mandibles" required inferior border anchorage to obtain adequate stability. The other extreme, that of a completely dense cortical mandible, required careful implant site preparation including tapping. These commonly found bone density variants guided surgical osteotomy preparation to diminish the possibility of adverse outcomes. These variants however, made it impossible to have a uniform data set for evaluation of implant treatment using All-on-Four immediate function.

Reported here are findings and results of treatment of 857 consecutive implants of which 428 were angulated. Representative case reports follow.

CASE REPORT I

A 75-year-old male patient presented with a diagnosis of a hopeless dentition due to severe periodontal disease (**Fig. 1**A). The past medical history was significant for well controlled Type II diabetes (A1c 6.8), hypertension, and hypercholesterolemia. He denied any drug allergies or history of smoking. His current medication included diltiazem hydrochloride 360 mg/day; lisinopril, 40 mg/day; metoprolol, 100 mg/day; glipizide, 10 mg/day; metformin, 300 mg/day; and aspirin, 81 mg /day. The surgical-restorative plan called for the removal of all remaining teeth, debridement of hard and soft tissue, mandibular alveolar reduction of 5 mm, and placement of mandibular implants using the All-on-Four technique.

The CBCT mandibular study revealed 70% to 90% bone loss on the remaining teeth without significant intrabony pathology. Approximately 14.5 mm were measured from the usable crest of the alveolus to the mental foramen bilaterally with no evidence of an exaggerated anterior IAN loop.

The intraoral examination revealed gross periodontal disease, attachment loss, and Class III mobility of the remaining teeth. The patient had been edentulous in the maxilla and partially edentulous in the mandible for 15 years. The maxillary complete denture had noticeable wear on the occluding surfaces of the mandibular anterior teeth with papillomatosis due to lack of proper fit of the prosthesis. The remaining mandibular anterior dentition had over-erupted and drifted, rendering unaesthetic diastemas and an uneven incisal plane suggesting combination syndrome. In addition, the patient had full-crown anterior tooth exposure while in repose. Bone reduction of 5 mm from the cement enamel junction of the incisors and 7 mm from the canines and first premolars was planned.

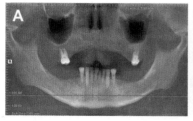 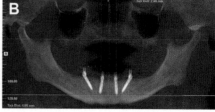

Fig. 1. (*A*) Preoperative cone beam CT scan showing compromised dentition. (*B*) Four-month postoperative iCAT study.

Surgical treatment was completed under IV sedation including intraoperative glucose monitoring. Teeth were removed via a periotome and forceps. Midcrestal incisions were made bilaterally from the retromolar pad to the midline within keratinized tissue. Inverse hockey incisions were made in the posterior to facilitate flap reflection. The mentalis muscle was partially reflected leaving 50% of the insertion intact. The mental nerve was identified bilaterally in relation to the distal most extraction sites. The alveolar bone shelf was prepared reducing bone level by 5 to 7 mm. The midline was identified and a 2 mm twist drill used to place the Malo guide. Posterior implant sites were developed just distal to the second premolar at 30° angles and the anterior sites at the canine-lateral incisor areas. All sites were prepared in a sequential fashion (without under preparation) using copious sterile saline irrigation. All implants placed were 4 × 18 mm NobelBiocare SpeedyGroovy RP with torque values of 45 Ncm.

Following fixture placement, straight or angulated multiunit abutments (NobelBiocare, Yorba Linda, CA, USA) were placed and torqued following manufacturer's instructions to allow for immediate prosthetic rehabilitation with fixed acrylic prostheses followed by soft tissue management and closure.

Multiunit impression copings were attached to the prosthetic abutments. An impression was made using a clear disposable tray using cartridge dispensed Aquasil Ultra Rigid Regular Set and Aquasil Ultra Deca (Dentsply Caulk, Milford, DE, USA). The impression was allowed to set, then removed and inspected for completeness. The impression was then poured using soft tissue material (Gigifast Ridgid, Zhermack Technical, Bovino, Italy) and type IV dental stone. Temporary cylinders were then connected to prosthetic abutments and luted to the mandibular complete denture using Trad (GC America, Aslip, IL, USA) acrylic resin verifying the occlusal plane orientation. The interim prosthesis was then finished on the surgical casts and delivered directly over the abutments, about 2.5 hours later. Prosthetic screws were torqued to 15 Ncm and access holes sealed with Teflon tape and Fermit (Ivoclar Vivadent AG, Liechtenstein). The occlusion of the prosthesis was designed in centric and group function. Patients were advised to eat only soft food for the first 4 months. The patient was seen for follow-up appointments after 10 days, 2 months, and 4 months. CBCT and periapical radiographs were obtained to evaluate bone healing around the dental implants (see **Fig. 1**B).

Final impressions were made after 4 months of healing. At that time, maxillomandibular records were obtained with a Denar Slidematic facebow (Whip-Mix Corp, Louisville, KY, USA) and ACU-flow Bite Registration Material (Great Lakes Prosthodontics Tonawanda, NY, USA). The interim prosthesis was removed and implant stability checked manually using a torque wrench. Angulated multiunit abutments were torqued to 15 Ncm and straight abutments to 35 Ncm. A Pattern Resin LS (GC America, Aslip, IL, USA) jig over temporary copings was fixed over corresponding implants and joined with resin. After setting, final impressions were made using Imprint 3 Monophase (Medium Body) and Imprint 3 Penta Heavy Body (3M ESPE, St Paul, MN, USA) impression materials on rigid disposable trays then poured with soft tissue material and type IV dental stone. Irreversible hydrocolloid (Jeltrate Plus, Dentsply, York, PA, USA) impressions were made of the maxillary and mandibular interim prostheses and poured in type III dental stone. Casts obtained from the interim prostheses were then articulated. The master casts were cross-mounted with the interim prosthesis in place while the patient waited in the dental chair. This technique allowed for recording of the patient's horizontal and vertical dimension of occlusion. The final prosthesis was made following NobelBiocare Procera bridge guidelines with a milled titanium framework. The occlusion was set in centric with group function for laterotrusive and protrusive excursions. The final prosthetic screws were torqued to 15 Ncm and access holes sealed with Teflon tape and composite resin. One-year postsurgical periapical radiographs were obtained and used to evaluate implant bone levels (**Fig. 2**).

CASE REPORT II

A 47-year-old female with a nonrestorable dentition due to severe decay and periodontal disease was treatment-planned for a full-mouth extraction, debridement of soft and hard tissue, alveolar shelf preparation, placement of implants using the All-on-Four immediate load technique, and delivery of an immediate upper denture. Past medical history was noncontributory except for a one pack per day, 25-year

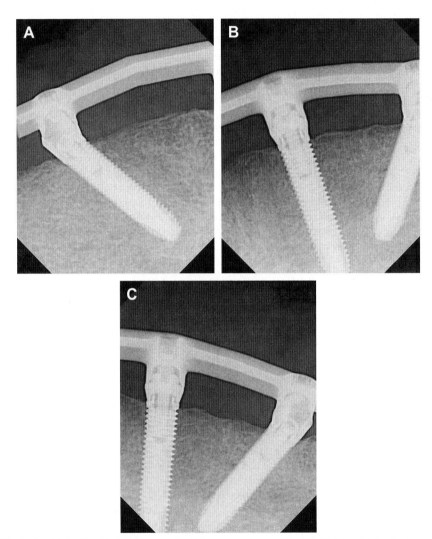

Fig. 2. (*A*) Right tilted implant bone level 1 year postoperative. (*B*) Right axial implant bone level 1 year postoperative. (*C*) Left axial and tilted implants bone levels 1 year postrestoration.

smoking history. Her physical examination was significant for multiple decayed and fractured teeth with severe periodontal disease. Intraoral soft tissues displayed typical findings of severe periodontal disease with the remaining teeth showing gross mobility and attachment loss.

The CBCT mandibular study revealed 80% bone loss on the remaining teeth with generalized chronic periapical abscesses (**Fig. 3**). Approximately 12 mm were measured from the usable crest of the alveolus to the mental foramen bilaterally. There was no evidence of an exaggerated anterior IAN loop.

The patient had been partially edentulous in both the maxilla and mandible for the last 20 years. The maxillary and mandibular remaining dentition exhibited generalized decay. The teeth were deemed hopeless. Bone reduction of 3 mm was planned.

The surgical procedure was completed under IV sedation. The remaining teeth and root remnants were surgically removed. Midcrestal incisions were made from the retromolar pads to the midline bilaterally with inverse distal hockey stick releases. Full-mucoperiosteal flaps were elevated lingually and labially with care to maintain keratinized tissue. The mental foramen was identified bilaterally with the dissection maintained on an equal plane of the foramen. With optimal visibility of the surgical field the extraction sites were debrided of necrotic tissue until only healthy bone was left. The All-on-Four bone shelf was developed at the predetermined level. Bone removed was saved for possible future use. A barrel acrylic bur under copious sterile saline irrigation was used to refine the bone shelf.

The midline was demarcated and distal implant sites prepared at a 30° angle. Anterior sites were developed in the lateral-canine region. Once all primary implant sites were verified as optimal for A-P spread the sites were enlarged with the 2 mm bur to a depth of 18 mm and guide pins were used to verify implant angulation. The 2.4/2.8 drills were used next to the appropriate depth. At this point the bone density was appreciated and all sites were further prepared with the 3 mm drill, except the distal sites were prepared to a depth of 13 mm. The anterior sites were further prepared with the 3.2/3.6 drill to a depth of 15 mm. Before placement all osteotomy sites

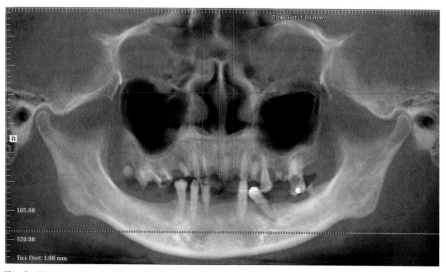

Fig. 3. Preoperative iCAT study showing rampant decay.

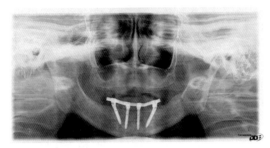

Fig. 4. One-year film showing titanium framework and stable restoration.

were irrigated. The implants were placed and torqued to 45 Ncm. Prosthetic abutments were placed and verified against the surgical guide. Wound closure was achieved with 3.0 chromic gut in an interrupted fashion after appropriate soft tissue management.

The same prosthetic procedures described in the previous case were followed following fixture placement. One year later periapical radiographs were obtained to evaluate bone level (**Fig. 4**).

CASE REPORT III

A 65-year-old female with a 40-year history of mandibular edentulism presented with a chief complaint of inability to wear her lower denture (**Fig. 5**). Her treatment plan called for placement of four implants with immediate loading using the All-on-Four technique. Her medical history was significant for allergy-induced asthma, arthritis, osteopenia, gastric reflux, depression, and chronic sinusitis. She did not report any known drug allergies and her medications consisted of Advair, two puffs daily; ProAir

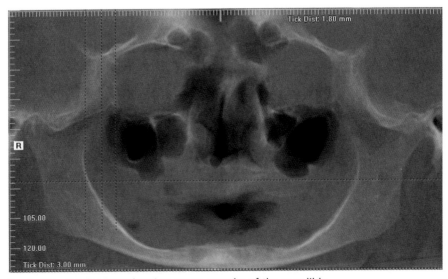

Fig. 5. Preoperative iCAT showing severe atrophy of the mandible.

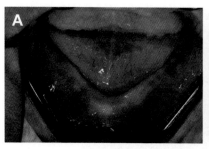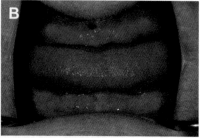

Fig. 6. (*A*) Occlusal view of the mandible showing severe loss of bone. (*B*) Avulsion of the floor of mouth 8–10 mm above the alveolar ridge.

as a rescue inhaler; omeprazole, 20 mg every day; Lexapro, 20 mg every day; alendronate, 70 mg once per week; multiple vitamins; and calcium supplements. Due to her history of bisphosphonate use she underwent a preoperative fasting collagen type I C-telopeptide blood test that was read as 150 pg/mL. The value was on the low range of the accepted threshold for surgery; therefore, she was kept off the medication for 6 months after surgery.

Her intraoral examination was significant for maxillary and mandibular edentulism with severe soft and hard tissue loss (**Fig. 6**A). The mandible displayed a thin band of keratinized tissue and the floor of mouth rose approximately 8 to 10 mm above the mandibular ridge at rest (see **Fig. 6**B). The mental nerves were palpable through the mucosa bilaterally and she displayed a V-shaped mandible. Her preoperative CBCT was reviewed for available bone height and mandibular anatomy. At the mental foramen region she displayed a total mandibular height of 6.90 mm on the right and 7.52 mm on the left. The symphysis displayed a height of 11.42 to 11.76 from right to left. On sagittal view, the mandible displayed a tubular anatomy with poorly defined marrow space devoid of trabecular bone.

Surgery was performed under IV sedation with appropriate monitoring. An inverse hockey stick incision was made in the retromolar region with continuation midcrestally around the arch. Care was used to stay within the keratinized soft tissue band. Full-mucoperiosteal flaps were developed with particular attention to the mental nerve and mentalis muscle insertion. The nerves were identified bilaterally and carefully distalized (**Fig. 7**). Posterior implant site preparation was then made through the mental

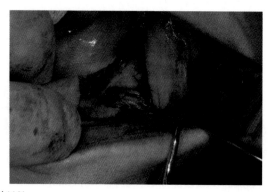

Fig. 7. Lateralized IAN.

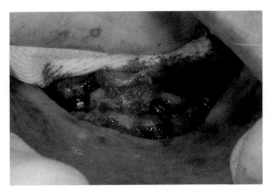

Fig. 8. Anterior implant placement using a V-4 configuration.

foramen bilaterally. Anterior sites were prepared in a "V" configuration (**Fig. 8**). All sites were prepared in a stepwise fashion under copious sterile saline irrigation to the inferior cortex. Distal sites were prepared to accommodate NobelBiocare Speedy Groovy implants 4 × 15 mm and the anterior 4 × 13 mm. Tapping was done to ensure passive fit. Final placement torque values were at or above 45 Ncm. After prosthetic abutment placement closure was completed with the aid of transosseous sutures to support muscle attachment and reposition the floor of the mouth. Prosthetic procedures then followed for delivery of the implant-supported fixed prosthesis.

Following scheduled postoperative and restorative appointments, a new maxillary complete denture was fabricated occluding against the mandibular final hybrid prosthesis (**Fig. 9**). Prosthetic teeth were arranged in bilateral balanced occlusion. Final prosthetic screws were torqued to 15 Ncm and access holes sealed with Teflon tape and composite resin. The 1-year postsurgical radiographs showed a very stable bone level at all implant sites regardless of axial or tilted position (**Fig. 10**).

RESULTS

During the course of 3 years, 219 patients were treated with mandibular All-on-Four immediate load. This diverse group of patients included dentate and edentulous patients as well as 64 smokers, 20 patients with diabetes, and 45 severe bruxers. The average age of this population was 60.95, including 98 males and 121 females. A total of 876 implants were placed and immediately loaded. Three implants failed to integrate, resulting in a success rate of 99.66%. The diabetes and bruxism groups did not experience any failures and only one implant was lost in the smoking group. There were two failures in the low-risk group.

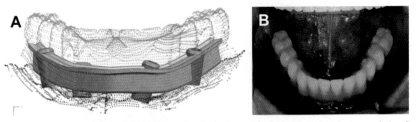

Fig. 9. (*A*) Final mandibular hybrid prosthesis design. (*B*) Clinical occlusal view of the final mandibular prosthesis.

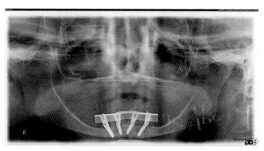

Fig. 10. Radiographic evaluation of the final prosthesis after 1 year of function.

Failure was defined as any implant demonstrating an inability to withstand 15 to 35 Ncm of torque at the fourth month postoperatively (**Table 1**). Of the three implants that did not achieve integration, two were axially placed and one tilted. During the treatment time there were no prostheses failures recorded, thus patients did not have to return to dentures. Of the 219 patients, 173 were transitioned into their final hybrid fixed prosthesis at the time of this article.

The failed implants succumbed late (after 8 weeks) and were thought to be caused by intraosseous infection because these failures occurred in patients who underwent concomitant extractions of teeth—demonstrating significant periapical pathology.

Nonintegrated implants were removed and new implants concomitantly placed into adjacent sites and then immediately loaded. The three failure cases were subsequently transitioned into final prostheses.

DISCUSSION

The technical factors that appear to have led to success in this study were careful implant site preparation including tapping, the use of relatively low torque-producing implants, and preparation of an All-on-Four shelf to provide interrestorative space and establish optimum implant sites. Additionally, the use of the V-4 technique in highly atrophic mandibles or nerve transposition to improve A-P spread, were also factors leading to successful All-on-Four therapy.

Table 1
Implant series life table

Axial Implant Life Table	Time (mo)	Patients	Implants Placed	Failed Implants	Interval Survival Rate (%)	Overall Survival Rate (%)
	0–2	219	438	2	99.54	99.54
	2–4	219	438	0	100.00	99.54
	4–12	219	438	0	100.00	99.54
	12–24	219	438	0	100.00	99.54
	24–36	219	438	0	100.00	
Tilted Implant Life Table	0–2	219	438	1	99.77	99.77
	2–4	219	438	0	100.00	99.77
	4–12	219	438	0	100.00	99.77
	12–24	219	438	0	100.00	99.77
	24–36	219	438	0	100.00	
Cumulative Survival Rate	0–36	219	876	3	99.66	99.66

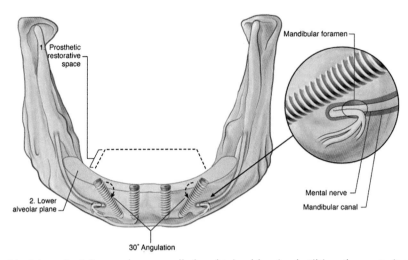

Fig. 11. Adequate A-P spread can usually be obtained by simply tilting the posterior implant. (*From* Jensen OT, Adams MW, Cottam JR, et al. The all on 4 shelf: mandible. J Oral Maxillofac Surg 2011;69:175–81; with permission.)

When the nerve was relatively anterior (**Fig. 11**) or an anterior loop was present (**Fig. 12**), distalization of the nerve was done using piezosurgery (**Fig. 13**). This allowed for placement of implants into more distal locations (**Fig. 14**). The use of transalveolar implant placement posterior to the mental foramen, done without disturbing the nerve, was another alternative used to increase A-P spread (**Figs. 15–18**).

The high success rate obtained in this series, including the finding of minimal periimplant bone loss, even when multiple extractions were done and bone reduction was required, may be the result of maximizing A-P spread. An A-P spread that minimizes distal cantilever and establishes a well distributed four-point stability probably contributed to both implant and prosthetic success.

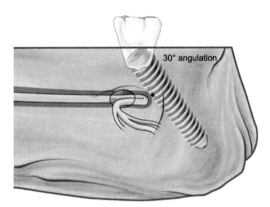

Fig. 12. The nerve will not need to be transposed if there is adequate alveolar height above the nerve to gain A-P spread. (*From* Jensen OT, Adams MW, Cottam JR, et al. The all on 4 shelf: mandible. J Oral Maxillofac Surg 2011;69:175–81; with permission.)

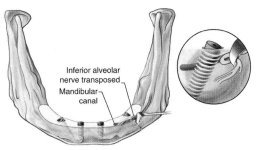

Fig. 13. By decortication laterally, the IAN can be transposed posteriorly to improve A-P spread when necessary. (*From* Jensen OT, Adams MW, Cottam JR, et al. The all on 4 shelf: mandible. J Oral Maxillofac Surg 2011;69:175–81; with permission.)

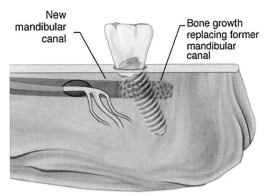

Fig. 14. With atrophy, the nerve presents higher toward the crest and may need to be distalized to gain adequate A-P spread with the implant being placed into the mental foramen. (*From* Jensen OT, Adams MW, Cottam JR, et al. The all on 4 shelf: mandible. J Oral Maxillofac Surg 2011;69:175–81; with permission.)

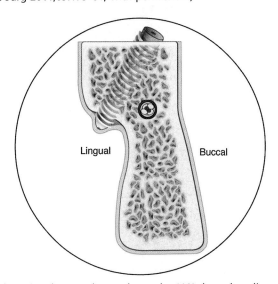

Fig. 15. Where there is adequate bone above the IAN, buccal to lingual (transalveolar) implant placement can be done. (*From* Jensen OT, Adams MW, Cottam JR, et al. The all on 4 shelf: mandible. J Oral Maxillofac Surg 2011;69:175–81; with permission.)

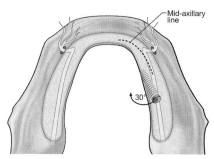

Fig. 16. Using a "flare angulation" of 30° combined with the distal 30° angle, the nerve can be avoided and fixation obtained in the lingual plate. (*From* Jensen OT, Adams MW, Cottam JR, et al. The all on 4 shelf: mandible. J Oral Maxillofac Surg 2011;69:175–81; with permission.)

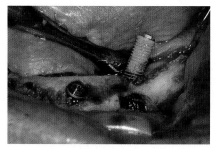

Fig. 17. A clinical example of transalveolar placement missing the nerve to engage into the lingual plate.

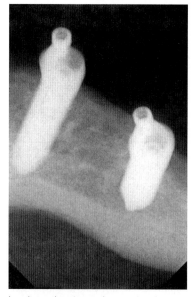

Fig. 18. Osseointegration develops despite a shorter implant used to gain favorable insertion torque for immediate function.

SUMMARY

Immediate function with Brånemark implants is well established for the mandible. This article describes a series of 857 implants placed consecutively in which very few implants failed or lost bone despite the dynamic healing conditions of simultaneous dental extractions and bone leveling. Though these findings are relatively early, 3 years or fewer, it appears that the immediate function All-on-Four procedure can be done with a high degree of confidence for the mandible—putting into question the need for additional implants.

REFERENCES

1. Brånemark PI, Hanso BO, Adell R, et al. Osseointegrated implants in the treatment of the edentulous jaw. Experience from a 10-year period. Scand J Plast Reconstr Surg Suppl 1977;16:1–132.
2. Brånemark PI, Zarb GA, Albrekson T, editors. Tissue-implanted prosthesis: osseointegration in clinical dentistry. Chicago: Quintessence; 1985.
3. Tada S, Strengoiu R, Kitamura E, et al. Influence of implant design and bone quality on stress/strain distribution in bone around implants: a 3-dimensional finite element analysis. Int J Oral Maxillofac Implants 2003;18:357–68.
4. Rangert B, Sullivan RM, Jemt T. Load factor control for implants in the posterior partially edentulous segment. Int J Oral Maxillofac Implants 1987;12:360–70.
5. Rangert B, Kroght PH, Langer B, et al. Bending overload and implant fracture: a retrospective clinical analysis [see comments]. Int J Oral Maxillofac Implants 1995;10(3):326–34 [published erratum appears in Int J Oral Maxillofac Implants 1996;11(5):575.].
6. Jensen OT, Nock D. Inferior alveolar nerve repositioning in conjunction with placement of osseointegrated implants: a case report. Oral Surg Oral Med Oral Pathol 1988;63(3):263–8.
7. Hirsch JM, Brånemark PI. Fixture stability and nerve function after transposition and lateralization of the inferior alveolar nerve and fixture installation. Br J Oral Maxillofac Surg 1995;33(5):276–81.
8. Jensen J, Reiche-Fischel O, Sindert-Peterson S. Nerve transposition and implant placement in the posterior atrophic mandibular alveolar ridge. J Oral Maxillofac Surg 1994;53(7):662–8.
9. Hashemi HM. Neurosensory function following mandibular nerve lateralization for placement of implants. Int J Oral Maxillofac Surg 2010;39:452–6.
10. Krekmanov LM, Kahn M. Tilting of posterior mandibular and maxillary implants for improved prosthesis support. Int J Oral Maxillofac Implants 2000;15(3):405–14.
11. Rangert BT, Jemt T. Forces and moments on Branemark implants. Int J Oral Maxillofac Implants 1989;4(3):241–7.
12. Bellini CM, Romeo D. A finite element analysis of tilted versus nontilted implant configurations in the edentulous maxilla. Int J Prosthodont 2000;22(2):155–7.
13. Bellini CM, Romeo D. Comparison of tilted versus nontilted implant-supported prosthetic designs for the restoration of the edentuous mandible: a biomechanical study. Int J Oral Maxillofac Implants 2000;24(3):511–7.
14. Testori T, Del Fabbro M, Capelli M, et al. Immediate occlusal loading and tilted implants for the rehabilitation of the atrophic edentulous maxilla. One-year interim results of a multicenter prospective study. Clin Implant Dent Relat Res 2008;19:227–32.

15. Capelli MF, Zuffetti F, Del Fabro M, et al. Immediate rehabilitation of the completely edentulous jaw with fixed prostheses supported by either upright or tilted implants: a multicenter clinical study. Int J Oral Maxillofac Implants 2007; 22(4):639–44.

16. Calandriello R, Tomatis T. Simplified treatment of the atrophic posterior maxilla via immediate/early function and tilted implants: a prospective 1-year clinical study. Clin Implant Dent Relat Res 2000;7(Suppl 1):S1–12.

17. Satoh T, Maed Y. Biomechanical rationale for intentionally inclined implants in the posterior mandible using 3D finite element analysis. Int J Oral Maxillofac Implants 2005;20(4):533–9.

18. Fortin Y, Sullivan RM. The Marius implant bridge: surgical and prosthetic rehabilitation for the completely edentulous upper jaw with moderate to severe resorption: a 5-year retrospective clinical study. Clin Implant Dent Relat Res 2002;4(2): 69–77.

19. Krekmanov L. Placement of posterior mandibular and maxillary implants in patients with severe bone deficiency: a clinical report of procedure. Int J Oral Maxillofac Implants 2000;15(5):722–30.

20. Aparicio C, Perales P, Ranger B. Tilted implants as an alternative to maxillary sinus grafting: a clinical, radiologic, and periotest study. Clin Implant Dent Relat Res 2001;3:39–49.

21. Aparicio C, Arevalo X, Ouzzani W, et al. A retrospective clinical and radiographic evaluation of tilted implants used in the treatment of the severely resorbed edentulous maxilla. Appl Osseointegration Res 2002;3:17–21.

22. Schnitman PA, Wohrle PS, Rubenstein JE, et al. Ten-year results for Branemark implants immediately loaded with fixed prostheses at implant placement. Int J Oral Maxillofac Implants 1997;12(4):495–503.

23. Gallucc GO, Bernard JP. Immediate loading with fixed screw-retained provisional restorations in edentulous jaws: the pickup technique. Int J Oral Maxillofac Implants 2000;19(4):524–33.

24. Ganeles J, Rosenberg MM. Immediate loading of implants with fixed restorations in the completely edentulous mandible: report of 27 patients from a private practice. Int J Oral Maxillofac Implants 2001;16(3):418–26.

25. De Bruyn H, Van De Velde T, Copllaert B. Immediate functional loading of TiO-blast dental implants in full-arch edentulous mandibles: a 3-year prospective study. Clin Oral Implants Res 2008;19:717–23.

26. Cooper LF, Rahman A, Moriarty J, et al. Immediate rehabilitation with endosseous implants: Simultaneous extraction, implant placement and loading. Int J Oral Maxillofac Implants 2002;17:517–25.

27. Grunder U. Immediate functional loading of immediate implants in edentulous arches: two-year results. Int J Periodontics Restorative Dent 2001;21:545–51.

28. Kacer CM, Dyer JD, Kraut RA. Immediate loading of dental implants in the anterior and posterior mandible: a retrospective study of 120 cases. J Oral Maxillofac Surg 2010;68:2861–7.

29. Gallucci GO, Morton D, Weber HP. Loading protocols for dental implants in edentulous patients. Int J Oral Maxillofac Implants 2009;24(Suppl 1):132–46.

30. Malo P, Rangert B, Nobre M. "All-on-four" immediate-function concept with the Branemark system implants for completely edentulous mandibles: a retrospective clinical study. Clin Implant Dent Relat Res 2003;5(Suppl 1):2–9.

31. Khatami AN, Smith CR. "All-on-Four" immediate function concept and clinical report of treatment of an edentulous mandible with a fixed complete denture and milled titanium framework. J Prosthodont 2008;17(1):47–51.

32. Jensen OT, Adams MW. All-on-4 Treatment of highly atrophic mandible with mandibular V-4: report of 2 cases. J Oral Maxillofac Surg 2009;67:1503–9.
33. Wegenberg BD, Ginsberg TR. Immediate implant placement with removal of the natural teeth: retrospective analysis of 1,081 implants. Compend Contin Educ Dent 2001;22:399–409.
34. Schwartz-Arad D, Chaushu G. Placement of implants into fresh extraction sites: 4 to 7 years retrospective evaluation of 95 immediate implants. J Periodontol 1997; 68(11):1110–6.
35. Tolman DE, Keller EE. Endosseous implant placement immediately following dental extraction and alveloplasty: preliminary report with 6-year follow-up. Int J Oral Maxillofac Implants 1991;6(1):24–8.
36. Evian CI, Emling R. Retrospective analysis of implant survival and the influence of periodontal disease and immediate placement on long-term results. Int J Oral Maxillofac Implants 2004;19(3):393–8.
37. Mensdorff-Pouilly N, Haas R, Mailath G, et al. The immediate implant: a retrospective study comparing the different types of immediate implantation. Int J Oral Maxillofac Implants 1994;9:571–8.
38. Villa R, Rangert B. Early loading of interforaminal implants immediately installed after extraction of teeth presenting endodontic and periodontal lesions. Clin Implant Dent Relat Res 2005;7(Suppl 1):528–35.
39. Cosci F, Cosci B. A 7-year retrospective study of 423 immediate implants. Compend Contin Educ Dent 1997;18:940–50.
40. Malo P, de Araujo Nobre M, Rangert B. Implants placed in immediate function in periodontally compromised sites: a five-year retrospective and one-year prospective study. J Prosthet Dent 2007;97(Suppl 6):S86–95 [erratum appears in J Prosthet Dent 2008;99(3):167].
41. Louble M, Maes F, Shutyer F. Assessment of bone segmentation quality of cone beam CT versus multi-slice spiral CT: a pilot study. Oral Surg Oral Med Oral Pathol Oral Radiol Endod 2006;120:225–34.
42. Suomalainen A, Vehmes T, Kortesniemi M. Accuracy of linear measurement using dental cone beam and coronal multislice computer tomography. Dentomaxillofac Radiol 2008;37:10–7.
43. Lofthag-Hansen S, Grondahl K, Ekestubbe A. Cone-beam CT for preoperative implant planning in the posterior mandible: visibility of anatomical landmarks. Clin Implant Dent Relat Res 2009;11:246–55.

Orthognathic and Osteoperiosteal Flap Augmentation Strategies for Maxillary Dental Implant Reconstruction

Ole T. Jensen, DDS, MS[a,b,*], Jason L. Ringeman, DDS, MD[c], Jared R. Cottam, DDS, MS[d], Nardy Casap, DMD, MD[e]

KEYWORDS

• Le Fort I • i-flap • Sub-Le Fort I • Interpositional bone graft

The use of vascularized osteotomies, particularly in orthognathic surgery is well founded in the literature.[1–6]

Edentulous total mandibular and maxillary osteotomies have also been reported.[7–11] In the last 10 years, the use of segmental osteotomies done with edentulous segments, including sandwich osteotomies, alveolar split osteotomies, and island bone flap approaches, have begun to be studied both in the laboratory and clinically.[7,12–19]

The advantage of alveolar osteotomies is that bone grafting is done interpositionally and crestal mucosal reflection is avoided, which generally leads to crestal bone stability, maintenance of gingival architecture, and a relatively uneventful recovery.

This article was previously published in the May 2011 issue of *Oral and Maxillofacial Surgery Clinics of North America*.

[a] Implant Dentistry Associates of Colorado, 8200 East Belleview Avenue, Suite 520E, Greenwood Village, CO 80111, USA

[b] Department of Oral and Maxillofacial Surgery, Hebrew University School of Dental Medicine, POB 12272, Jerusalem, 91120, Israel

[c] Tissue Engineering Institute of Colorado, 8200 East Belleview Avenue, Suite 520E, Greenwood Village, CO 80111, USA

[d] Private Practice, 15515 3rd Avenue, #E, Burien, WA 98166, USA

[e] Department of Oral and Maxillofacial Surgery, Faculty of Dental Medicine, Hebrew University, Hadassah, Jerusalem, Israel

* Corresponding author. Implant Dentistry Associates of Colorado, 8200 East Belleview Avenue, Suite 520E, Greenwood Village, CO 80111.

E-mail address: ole.jensen@clearchoice.com

Dent Clin N Am 55 (2011) 813–846
doi:10.1016/j.cden.2011.07.011
0011-8532/11/$ – see front matter © 2011 Elsevier Inc. All rights reserved.

Although only 2 long-term clinical studies have been reported using sandwich osteotomy bone grafting for implants, it seems that volumetric stability of the bone around later-placed implants is nearly equal to that of the native bone when implants are placed after osteotomy healing has occurred.[12,20]

In this article, 5 variations in orthognathic surgery procedures used to gain bone mass for implants are discussed: Le Fort I downgraft, Le Fort I distraction, the sub–Le Fort I interpositional sandwich graft, the segmental sandwich graft, and the island osteoperiosteal flap (i-flap) approach.

LE FORT I DOWNGRAFT

The use of iliac bone grafting for the Le Fort I downgraft is used to gain not only vertical dimension but also horizontal width.[21] The sinus floor can also be grafted such that after healing, usually 6 months for graft consolidation and up to 6 months for implant healing, implants can be placed for a fixed restoration as shown in **Figs. 1–10**.[22]

The technique involves making a vestibular incision and horizontal osteotomy cuts after elevation of the sinus membranes bilaterally through lateral window access (see **Fig. 5**). The pterygoid sutures and nasal septum are freed, and the maxilla is downfractured in a standard manner. However, because of severe atrophy, the maxilla often spontaneously fragments, so care must be taken when compared with younger dentate patients undergoing the Le Fort I procedure.

Following downfracture, the maxilla is mobilized forward using disimpaction forceps and then repositioned and bone plated in down and forward positions (see **Fig. 6**). A general rule of thumb is ten mm forward and ten mm downward. Fixation provides a very large interpositional graft zone for bone grafting. Grafting proceeds by first grafting the sinus floor with particulate marrow and then the anterior nasal floor, followed by block mortising and overgrafting the bone-plated regions to gain width (see **Fig. 7**). Consideration should be given to using resorbable bone plates, so that when implants are placed later, there will be no fixation screw interference. Once the graft is in place, which entails the combination of particulated bone marrow deep and corticocancellous blocks fixed with screws as overgraft, the wound is closed in 2 layers with slowly resorbing suture material. There should be no tension on the wound. Placement of a provisional denture at this time is a matter of judgment. When a denture is flangeless and borne only by the palate and crestal bone, and the confidence in the fixation is good, most often a denture can be placed early without

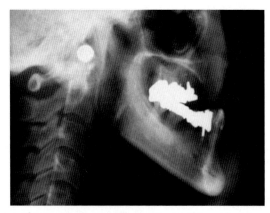

Fig. 1. Cephalogram of preoperative maxillary retrognathia and severe atrophy.

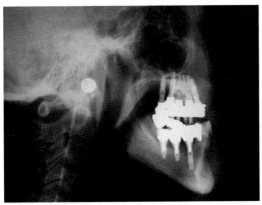

Fig. 2. Cephalogram posttreatment showing the maxilla in an anteriorized position with implants supporting a fixed restoration.

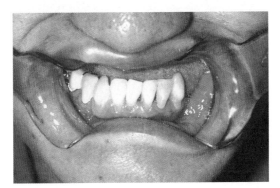

Fig. 3. Preoperative view intraorally with the absence of anterior projection of the maxilla.

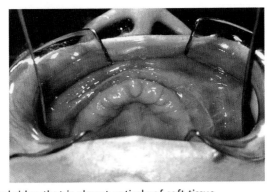

Fig. 4. The residual ridge that is almost entirely of soft tissue.

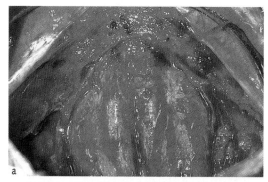

Fig. 5. Downfracture of the maxilla after elevation of the sinus membrane.

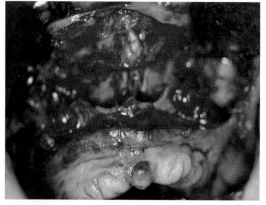

Fig. 6. Interpositional grafting space after fixation of the maxilla that was brought down 10 mm and forward 10 mm.

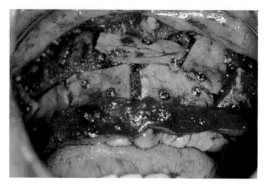

Fig. 7. Iliac marrow was used in the sinus floors and blocked fixed as overgraft.

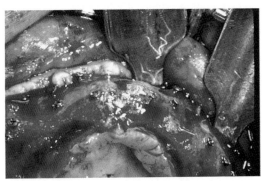

Fig. 8. Good consolidation with some areas of resorption on exposure of the maxilla 6 months later.

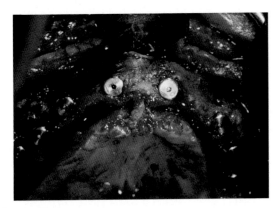

Fig. 9. Implant placement.

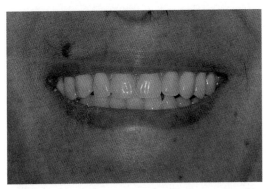

Fig. 10. Final restoration using a fixed denture prosthesis supported by 8 osseointegrated implants. A 10-year follow-up showed a stable graft and stable prosthesis.

risking wound dehiscence. On the other hand, when the Le Fort fixation is tenuous or the augmentation procedure opposes natural dentition, perhaps in a patient with bruxism, the use of a provisional denture should be curtailed.

Six months later, an incision is made 3 to 4 mm palatal of the alveolar crest around the arch (see **Fig. 8**). The flap is developed and lateralized to gain fixed connective tissue buccally after implants are placed and abutments are connected (see **Fig. 9**). Often, because implants are placed at this time, the bone is still not completely consolidated, although there is great variation between patients. When implants are firmly torqued into place, a 1-stage protocol is used; if not, a staged method.

Following osseointegration, the final fixed denture prosthesis is inserted, which is needed to support the lip and make up for still remaining jaw bone deficiency despite bone graft augmentation (see **Fig. 10**).

The advantage of the Le Fort I downgraft is a greatly increased bone mass available for osseointegration; but the disadvantage is that alveolar height may not be achieved and the position of the maxilla is never ideal, often being 5 to 10 mm retropositioned, despite advancement. Also, these cases require a lot of bone graft material, often necessitating posterior hip harvest.[23] Grafts can be expanded with allografts or alloplasts, but this may add additional risk for infection if the graft site becomes exposed.[24] The greatest disadvantage is the need for a secondary harvest site, which is not always possible in the elderly or in patients with back and extremity osteoarthritis.[25]

Therefore, the procedure may be relatively contraindicated in those older than 60 years, unless the patient is in excellent health, which suggests a great need to treat these not uncommonly found atrophic findings with an alternative method such as the use of bone morphogenetic protein 2 (BMP-2).

The use of BMP-2 for the Le Fort I procedure, however, is still in development. **Figs. 11–21** show a case in which BMP-2 was placed following downward and forward maxillary repositioning using a Le Fort I osteotomy in which sinus elevation was done. Although a large amount of BMP-2 on collagen sponge (only) was used, the resultant bone mass gain with this technique was much less than that found with iliac graft reconstruction, although sufficient to place 10-mm implants (see **Fig. 20**). The bone quality was excellent and osseointegration uneventful.

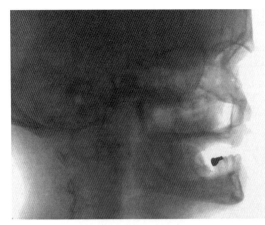

Fig. 11. Severe bone loss that resulted from the removal of upper teeth in a female patient with bruxism.

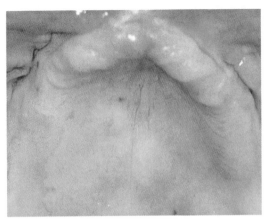

Fig. 12. Presentation of the maxilla as flat without much vestibule by 1-year postextraction.

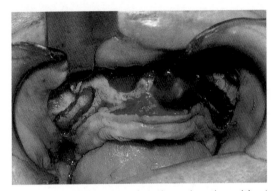

Fig. 13. Bilateral sinus membrane elevations done in conjunction with a Le Fort I distraction.

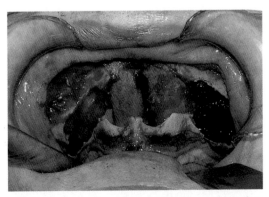

Fig. 14. Downfracturing the maxilla after osteotomy, preserving nasal and sinus membranes.

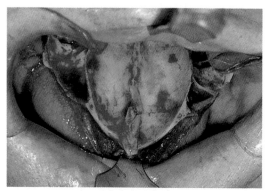

Fig. 15. The atrophied maxilla in the downfractured position.

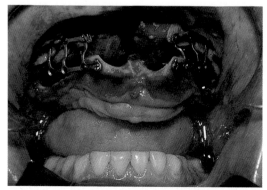

Fig. 16. Fixation with the maxilla down 10 mm and forward 10 mm in preparation for placement of BMP-2 graft.

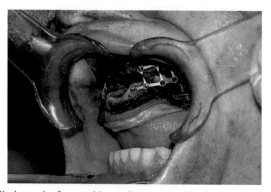

Fig. 17. The maxilla brought forward into alignment with the lower arch.

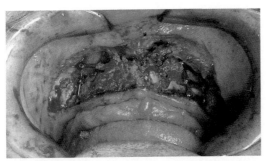

Fig. 18. Interpositional grafting done with BMP-2 and collagen sponge.

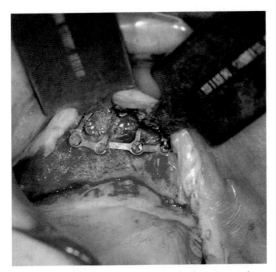

Fig. 19. The jaw exposed and fixation plates removed after 6 months.

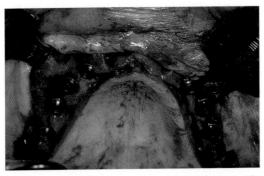

Fig. 20. Implant installation proceeded, but only implants that are 10 to 11.5 mm can be placed.

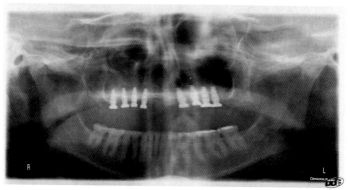

Fig. 21. Panorex showing implants. There is a modest volume of BMP-2 interpositional graft on the implants.

The grafting technique using BMP-2 is similar to iliac graft placement with the fragmented collagen sponges packed into the sinus floor first and then into the nasal floor, laterally around the osteotomy site, and into the wound closed primarily (see **Fig. 18**). When expansion of the graft is needed, the use of 20% to 30% demineralized freeze-dried bone allograft is advised. A large graft of BMP-2 requires 6 to 9 months for consolidation (see **Fig. 19**), although implants can be placed earlier into what feels like osteoid in a submerged approach. Exposure of implants is done with a palatal crestal bias to gain fixed connective tissue, and then the case may be restored with a fixed denture prosthesis.

Once again, the use of BMP-2 does not generally create an ideal reposition of the maxilla but does gain sufficient bone mass for dental implantation (see **Fig. 21**). The use of allograft as an expander has recently been shown to preserve the volume of the BMP-2 graft and should be considered in large graft sites.[26]

LE FORT I DISTRACTION

When there is adequate alveolar width for implants but the edentulous maxilla is in a retrognathic position, the maxilla can be distracted forward and downward to optimize prosthetics for implants, which must be placed secondarily. The great advantage of the distraction procedure is prosthodontist-directed repositioning of the maxilla into optimal position for emergence profile implant restoration. The surgeon unfamiliar with this procedure must understand that the edentulous jaw can be placed within 1 mm of the desired anterior maxillary alveolar position. For a retrodisplaced maxilla, Le Fort I distraction is the most accurate of all grafting or distraction approaches for gaining an esthetic emergence of an implant restoration.

The technique has limited use because it is a special situation approach for treating young female edentulous patients who present with a modest retropositioned maxilla that needs to be brought down and forward to bring the alveolus into orthoalveolar form to optimize perioral and gingival esthetics.[27]

The technique (**Figs. 22–27**) can be done in the office setting under intravenous anesthesia but is best done in the operating room. Medical models can be made from computerized axial tomography scan images and used to do mock Le Fort I surgery and distraction plate placement. The distraction plates are prebent and placed on the models to gain the appropriate vector for advancement, so they are ready for use during surgery.

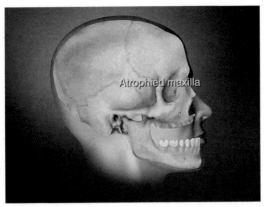

Fig. 22. The atrophied maxilla presenting as a retrodisplaced maxilla with vertical dimension loss.

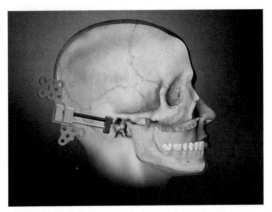

Fig. 23. Preparation for placement of a distraction bone plate by a Le Fort osteotomy along the area marked by the red line.

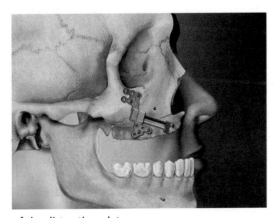

Fig. 24. Placement of the distraction plate.

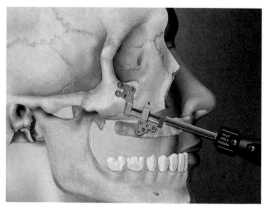

Fig. 25. The distraction can proceed 20 mm or more forward with a downfractured vector, gaining 10 mm of vertical.

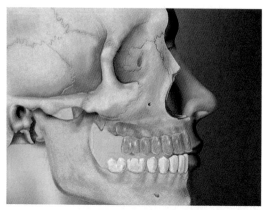

Fig. 26. With the maxilla in an idealized position, implant placement can proceed using a "gum-set" guide stent.

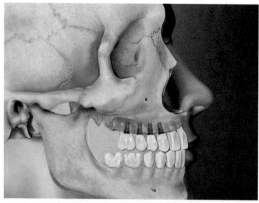

Fig. 27. Placement of posterior implants, leaving the incisors as pontics to develop emergence esthetics in the restoration.

Figs. 28–38 show the Le Fort I distraction technique. A vestibular incision is made in a 35-year-old female patient (see **Figs. 28** and **29**), and sinus membranes are elevated bilaterally followed by horizontal osteotomy cuts (see **Fig. 30**). The pterygoid sutures and nasal septum were freed using osteotomes, and then the maxilla is minimally downfractured to allow for freedom of movement. In the operating room, the maxilla can be fully mobilized, although this is not always necessary for unimpeded distraction to proceed. The distraction plates were then fixed into place with downward and medial vectors (see **Figs. 30** and **31**), with the osteotomy site open about 2 mm (see **Fig. 32**). The sinus floor was grafted but not the osteotomy sites. The distraction proceeded over a 2-week period following a 1-week latency (see **Figs. 33** and **34**). The use of BMP-2 as graft material not only facilitates sinus floor augmentation but also augments distraction osteogenesis, which to a great extent is based biologically on mechanoreceptor-induced BMP-2 signaling.[28]

The maxilla had healed well 6 months later. The bone plates were removed and implants placed transgingivally (see **Figs. 35** and **36**). And then, the final restoration was done (see **Figs. 37** and **38**), which showed a natural gingival emergence that was stable at 3 years.

SUB–LE FORT I INTERPOSTIONAL GRAFT

The long-span interpositional bone grafting of the maxilla, essentially a sub–Le Fort I sandwich osteotomy, can extend from the first molar to the first molar around the arch (**Figs. 39–46**).[29–34] When done in conjunction with sinus membrane elevation and BMP-2 grafting, a fair amount of bone mass can be obtained 6 to 9 months later. Multiple implants are usually placed for fixing provisionally as shown in **Fig. 44**.

The technique uses a horizontal vestibular incision from the first molar to the first molar around the arch. Sinus membranes are elevated from a lateral osteotomy approach. Then, using a curved saw blade, a horizontal osteotomy is made cutting through the lateral maxilla and then transsinus through the palatal vault just lateral of the nasal wall. Anteriorly, the anterior nasal spine is identified, and the alveolar bone cut is made beneath the nasal floor to connect with the posterior cuts. The maxilla is then freed with an osteotome usually spontaneously fracturing the area of the first molar in front of the tuberosity region. The maxilla pivots down in a kind of hinge movement creating a gap of up to 10 mm in what is essentially an extended

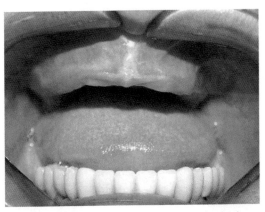

Fig. 28. Moderate vertical atrophy in a 35-year-old woman who had worn a denture for less than 10 years.

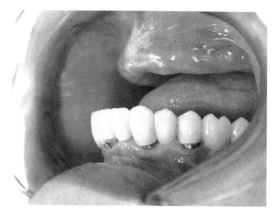

Fig. 29. Posterior displacement of the horizontal portion of the maxilla, making an ideal esthetic restoration impossible.

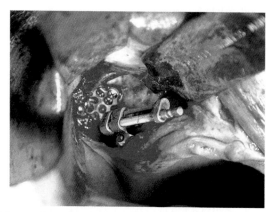

Fig. 30. A Le Fort I procedure was done and bone plates placed.

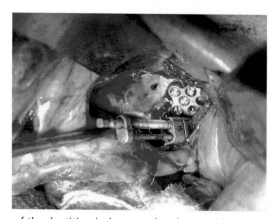

Fig. 31. The vector of the dentition is downward and toward the midline.

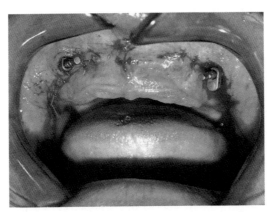

Fig. 32. After closure, the activation arms of the distracters are easily accessible in the vestibule. The denture flange is trimmed to avoid impingement.

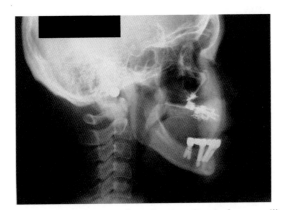

Fig. 33. A cephalogram with distraction plates in place but before maxillary advancement.

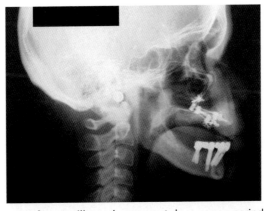

Fig. 34. A cephalogram after maxillary advancement done over a period of 2 weeks during which the maxilla was advanced 13 to 15 mm.

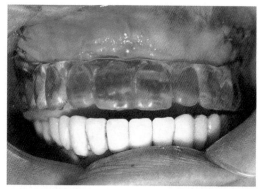

Fig. 35. The maxilla 6 months later after device removal with the implant guide stent in place.

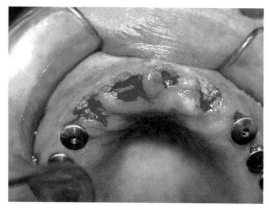

Fig. 36. Implant placement posteriorly and soft tissue sculpting interiorly.

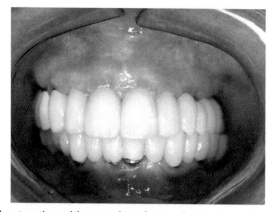

Fig. 37. The final restoration with natural teeth over denture emergence.

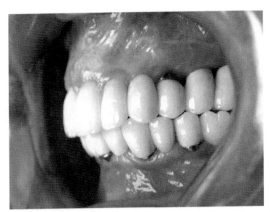

Fig. 38. Anterior projection seems normal, although gingival recession developed posteriorly by 3 years.

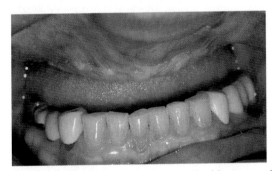

Fig. 39. Flat maxilla against a natural dentition in a 73-year-old woman who had a history of clenching.

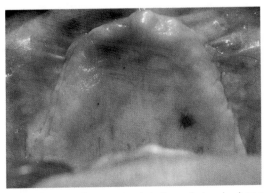

Fig. 40. Absence of a vestibule and near-complete loss of alveolar bone.

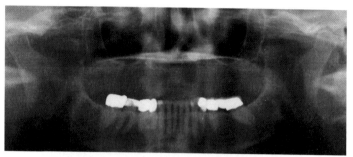

Fig. 41. Preoperative panorex.

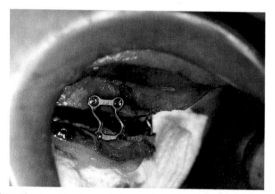

Fig. 42. Maxilla downfractured minimally in a sub–Le Fort I procedure.

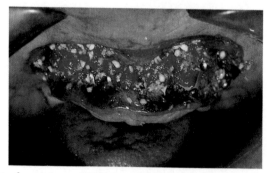

Fig. 43. Placement of a mixture of BMP-2 and 20% allograft following bone plating.

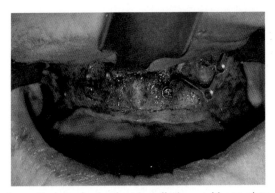

Fig. 44. Exposure 6 months later for implant installation and bone plate removal.

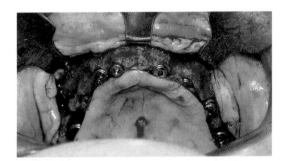

Fig. 45. Placement of implants.

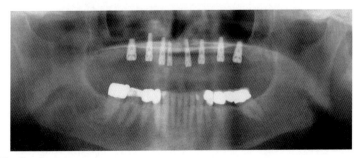

Fig. 46. Postimplant panorex.

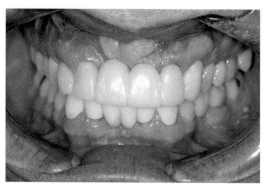

Fig. 47. One week post–sandwich osteotomy with a temporary bridge placed on 4 abutment teeth.

alveolar segmental sandwich (horseshoe) osteotomy (see **Fig. 42**). This sub–Le Fort I approach allows for the development of height but not the improvement of anterior posterior maxillary position. The segment is bone plated to a 10-mm interpostional gap that is then grafted with BMP-2 with a 20% allograft mix (see **Fig. 43**). The wound is then closed primarily and denture adjusted as needed.

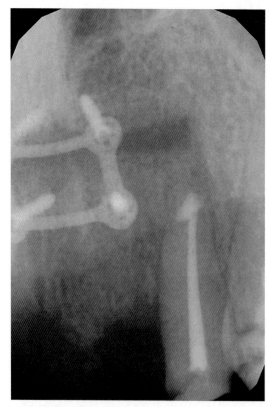

Fig. 48. On the day of surgery, sandwich osteotomy fixation with about a 4-mm vertical movement shown on the left.

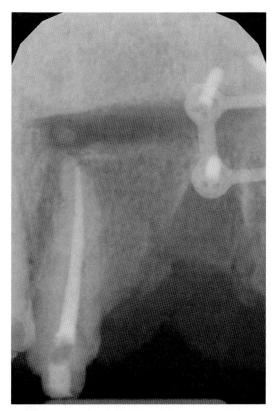

Fig. 49. Right side vertical movement close to 5 mm.

After 6 to 9 months, through a crestal incision, bone plates are removed and implants placed in a submerged protocol (see **Figs. 44–46**). Four months after placement, the implants are exposed and the final restoration is done.

This technique is very easily performed in an office setting using intravenous anesthesia. Elderly patients tolerate it well, and osseointegration develops from the

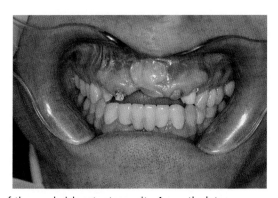

Fig. 50. Healing of the sandwich osteotomy site 4 months later.

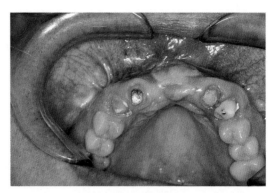

Fig. 51. Four months later, the lateral incisors and left canine are scheduled for removal.

interpositional graft. The disadvantage of the technique is that as the segment pivots downward in a hinge action, the anterior projection of the maxilla actually becomes more retrodisplaced. Also, the technique does nothing for gaining alveolar width that is often needed in these settings.

SANDWICH OSTEOTOMY

The short-span vertically deficient alveolus can often be corrected with a simple sandwich osteotomy. This osteotomy is especially beneficial in the maxillary esthetic zone.

When anterior teeth are to be lost because of caries or periodontal disease, especially if consecutive teeth are to be removed, a significant vertical defect will result despite socket preservation bone grafting. One way to correct this problem is to perform a sandwich osteotomy that includes the later-to-be-extracted teeth. By performing this osteotomy, the maxillary segment can be brought into a more ideal position, so that when dental extractions are done later, immediate implants can be placed and often times immediately temporized in preparation for a more ideal restoration.

Shown in **Figs. 47–55** is a 33-year-old man who traumatically lost the upper left central and lateral incisors, which was followed by a 6-tooth conventional bridge. Abutment teeth later failed necessitating removal of the central and lateral incisor and the left canine. Before removal of these teeth, however, a provisional bridge

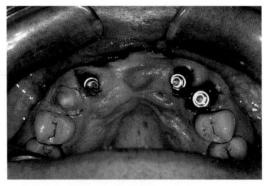

Fig. 52. Placement of implants after removal of the teeth.

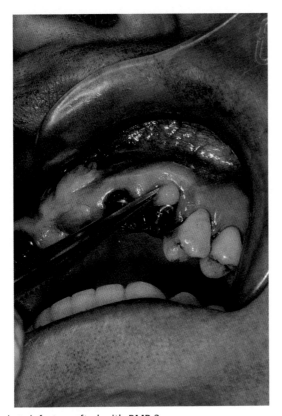

Fig. 53. Large socket defects grafted with BMP-2.

was made, and a sandwich osteotomy from the right canine to the left lateral incisor was performed, bringing down the segment 4 mm with interpositional bone grafting using BMP-2 (see **Figs. 47–50**). The temporary bridge was then retrofitted into place on the day of surgery (see **Fig. 47**). Four months later, the site had healed and the dental extractions were done. Implants were placed about 4 mm below the marginal gingiva and BMP-2 used for socket graft material (see **Figs. 51–55**). The provisional bridge was then retrofitted into place on the 3 implants and the right canine tooth (**Fig. 56**). A final bridge was placed 4 months later.

The experienced surgeon recognizes immediately the advantage of such a treatment plan in that no full flap is reflected; the crestal bone is relatively stable, extraction site grafting is a minimal risk variable, and immediate implant placement and temporization are well within the realm of effective procedures. But the major effect of this type of treatment is esthetic control of the alveolar plane and therefore the lack of the need for gingivoalveolar modification by hard and soft tissue grafting. The sandwich graft can be done consistently, especially in larger segments of 4 teeth or more.

The disadvantage of sandwich grafting is lack of people with experience and technical expertise. Those surgeons facile with orthognathic surgery should be able to perform the procedure without mishap, but careless surgery resulting in a torn pedicle can cause the complete loss of the segment, the soft issue, and all.

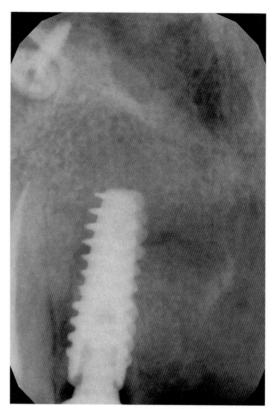

Fig. 54. Postimplant placement radiograph of the right side.

Sandwich grafting is not a good choice when the alveolar ridge is thin, perhaps 4 mm or less, because it does not improve alveolar width.

Depending on the interpositional graft material and the blood supply in the interpostional zone, healing can be variable but consolidation of the graft is usually quite firm by 4 months. The use of a barrier membrane is not required with the technique, although this is recommended with the use of alloplasts or allograft. In any case, it is advisable to place implants through the graft zone into basal bone to gain primary stability in cortical bone.

THE I-FLAP

The i-flap is a vascularized facial plate segment that is separated from basal bone for mobilization to gain alveolar width and some height. It is most frequently used in the maxilla for narrow-width segmental zones, usually of 2 or more teeth in length. It is possible to perform a full-arch i-flap procedure in the maxilla. In the mandible, caution should be used for alveolar splitting because the periosteum can easily detach.

The technique is done through an unreflected crestal incision in which an alveolar split osteotomy is done (book flap); the bone fragment is then separated from the basal bone (i-flap) but still remains attached to the periosteum to gain alveolar width following interpositional grafting.

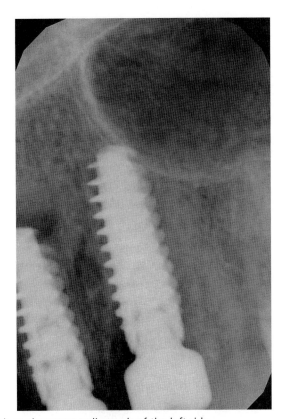

Fig. 55. Postimplant placement radiograph of the left side.

Figs. 57–62 shows an anterior deficient maxilla that was treated with i-flap alveolar expansion using BMP-2. Note the maintenance of plate thickness of the i-flap despite remodeling shrinkage in the interpostional graft zone 5 months after surgery. Implants were then placed for a fixed anterior bridge.

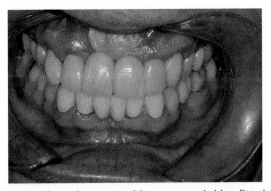

Fig. 56. One week postimplant placement with temporary bridge fitted to implants and 1 tooth abutment.

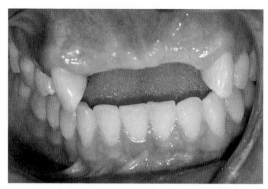

Fig. 57. A thin anterior maxilla that was treated by alveolar split bone grafting.

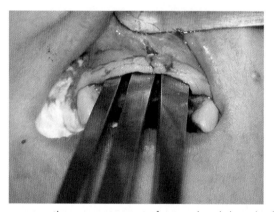

Fig. 58. After piezosurgery, the segment was outfractured and then the facial plate mobilized as an i-flap.

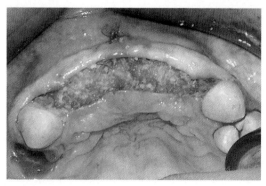

Fig. 59. Interplate grafting.

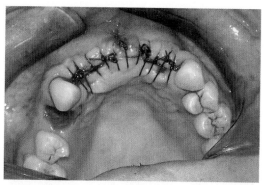

Fig. 60. The i-flap was advanced crestally to gain primary wound closure.

The advantage of an i-flap approach is the use of a mobilized, but still vascularized, buccal bone plate. This is especially useful in the maxilla, which resorbs facial plate in deference to palatal plate.[35] Essentially, by splitting the residual palatal bone and transferring the split fragment buccally, alveolar width is restored and a mature bone plate becomes available for protection of later-placed implants.

The preferred thickness of an i-flap is 2 mm or more to maintain plate integrity.[36] When i-flaps are thin, such as 1 mm thick, they can fully resorb, although they may still undergo replacement resorption without the loss of width gain from the expansion

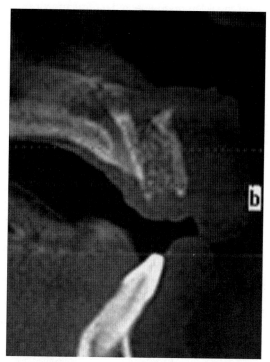

Fig. 61. Posttreatment computerized axial tomography scan showing graft site and width gain.

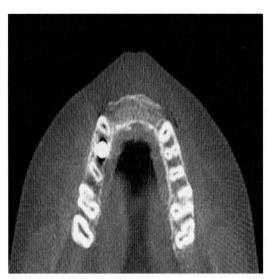

Fig. 62. Posttreatment computerized axial tomography scan showing anterior projection.

procedure.[37] The long-term consequence of using i-flaps for alveolar split sites is still uncertain. In one study, bone resorption developed within 2 years after placement of implants in a small percentage of sites treated, but accurate methods for determining buccal bone loss are lacking unless full flap exposure is done as a follow-up.[17]

The disadvantage of the i-flap approach is the requirement of technical skill to do what is essentially a blind technique. Also, the usual way to do an i-flap procedure is without rigid fixation, so suturing becomes the method of immobilization.

One advantage of the i-flap approach over the book flap approach is wound closure and vertical displacement of the facial plate because of the capacity for vertical movement of the bone fragment within a mobilized soft tissue flap, which can especially be helpful in posterior segmental i-flaps that can be advanced crestally to entirely close the wound even as 4 to 5 mm in width is obtained.

The i-flap approach can take the place of guided bone regeneration with much less operative time, less cost, limited risk of infection, and excellent healing potential. However, dimensional stability still needs to be addressed in the long term.[38]

DISCUSSION

The use of interpositional bone grafts with various jaw osteotomies and the smaller segmental osteoperiosteal flaps is becoming more commonly prescribed in the edentulous setting for augmentation and implant site preparation. The sandwich osteotomy, used in the posterior mandible, generally outperforms distraction osteogenesis and blocks bone grafting or guided bone regeneration.[19] Although posterior augmentation with titanium mesh has been successfully done using iliac particulate graft, en bloc iliac bone can resorb more than 50%.[39,40] The use of mesh protected morphogen grafting shows great promise but is still under development.[12,41] The osteotomy approach, preserving a vascular pedicle, often gains 8 to 10 mm in the posterior mandible, whereas guided bone regeneration only achieves modest vertical gains.[42] Monocortical blocks have been shown to have about a 5% early loss of the entire graft with up to 40% loss of graft volume because of late-term remodeling or inadequate consolidation.[43]

Stable results occur in the maxilla with osteoperiosteal flaps, such as with the sandwich osteotomy, especially for the esthetic zone. In this region, gingivoalveolar form is easier to obtain by the sandwich osteotomy bone grafting, moving segments down 5 mm or more to level of the alveolar plane. Reconstructing and leveling the alveolar plane corrects the common deformity found from periodontal bone loss.[17] This correction is more difficult to do with block grafting because resorption also can occur in the anterior maxilla, sometimes up to 40% by 1 year.[43,44] And when block grafts are lost in the anterior maxilla, the consequence is often a worsened defect, with disturbed healing potential for further attempts at reconstruction. The sandwich approach is more stable with less resorption at the crest, provided there is adequate width to the caudal segment. The interpositional graft technique eliminates the need for vertical alveolar distraction in most cases, limiting the use of distraction to vertical movements of 10 mm or more.[45]

Full-arch alveolar atrophy of the mandible and maxilla can often be treated without augmentation grafting by using All-on-Four technology and/or computer guided implant strategies.[46] The edentulous maxilla with severe atrophy can almost always be treated with an M4 technique, the letter "M" designating implant placement angulations when viewed on panorex.[47] When implants are placed at 30°, structures such as the sinus and nasal cavity are avoided, often circumventing the need to perform bone grafting. However, when the maxilla is extremely resorbed, a Le Fort I downgraft procedure is indicated.

The Le Fort I interpositional graft procedure must be contrasted with the more commonly done onlay grafting procedure.[47] Although onlay procedures have shown success, especially when combined with sinus floor grafting, the advantage of a Le Fort I downgraft is maxillary repositioning into a more biomechanically advantageous implant platform.[48] The onlay, onlay plus sinus floor graft, and Le Fort I interpositional graft variations have all shown very favorable implant success rates when done using a delayed implant placement strategy; but a repositioned maxilla always has less anterior cantilever. The use of simultaneous implant placement combined with maxillary repositioning has also been reported but requires adequate bone mass for fixation and is now infrequently done.[49] Two decades ago surgeons made the determination to delay implant placement in large iliac bone graft reconstructions of the maxilla. Implant success rates subsequently increased by 10% to 15%, approaching the success rate found in native bone.[50–52]

The final frontier of pedicled bone grafting, first biologically established by Bell and colleagues[4,5,53] nearly 40 years ago, is the development of small segment bone manipulations done in preparation for dental implant reconstruction. This is most clearly demonstrated in the alveolar split procedure in which the medullary blood supply is inconsequential and the periosteal vascular pedicle is the most significant contributor to osseous healing.[51] A rabbit tibia model determined that a thin pedicled segment separated from the tibial shaft by interpositional graft material remained vital with just periosteal blood supply.[53] However, overstripping of the bone leads to ischemia and osteocyte cell death on bone margins unattached to vascular supply.[53]

Another animal study compared interpositional grafting in split sites simultaneously with dental implant placement.[54] Immediately placed implants did not osseointegrate consistently when compared with distracted split sites with delayed placement, which indicates embarrassed vascular healing capacity from medullary blood flow disruption but also may indicate disturbance in periosteal hemodynamics. The exact nature of recovery of vascularity after alveolar split osteotomy is uncertain and requires study. Therefore, the installation of implants at the time of alveolar split should be done with caution.

It does seem intuitive that the smaller the segment, the less thick the bone plate being moved, the more tenuous the blood supply. In addition, the edentulous alveolus that results from the loss of teeth and diminished intramedullary blood supply may be more dependent on the periosteum than is generally understood.[55] For example, in one study, angiography was done in the mandible of middle age patients. Complete occlusion of the inferior alveolar vascular supply was discovered in 55% of patients studied.[56] These patients had almost no intraosseous vascular supply. This athero-sclerotic effect may not be as much of an issue in the maxilla because of collateral circulation but must nevertheless be considered a factor in confronting the aging population, affecting the design and execution of osteoperiosteal flaps.

The buccal plate is fragile, and splitting it away from the alveolus after full flap reflection has been shown both clinically and in animal studies to lead to complete plate resorption.[57,58] In one animal study, in which alveolar width distraction was done after full flap exposure of the site, complete resorption of the buccal plate occurred despite bone forming from the distraction procedure interpositionally.[58] Such may be the case clinically in full-flapped alveolar split cases that are grafted interpositionally.[17] The interpositional graft works adequately, but the buccal plate resorbs away. This finding was found in one case in which on reentry after anterior maxillary split grafting, much of the buccal plate was found to have resorbed away despite osseointegration occurring in the interpostional graft zone. The split graft, when reviewed photographically, had zones that were from 1 to 4 mm in thickness. Wherever the plate thickness was less than 2 mm, the plate had resorbed away.[17] Because of this type of evidence, still needing further substantiation, both clinically and in the laboratory, the development of periosteal attached bone fragment manipulation is advocated.

The challenge for the oral and maxillofacial surgeon in dental implant site preparation is to use judgment and skill, guided by biologic principles for alveolar reconstruction. Modest gains of 5 mm or less in width and height are often highly significant and usually extremely stable. The surgeon knows from orthognathic surgery that small precise osteotomy movements, well fixed, heal without significant relapse.[59] This experience in the dentate setting may not be fully achieved in parallel for the edentulous patient, but the use of an osteoperiosteal flap approach, perhaps mildly overcorrected to allow for reductive remodeling, should enhance outcome for the challenge of reconstruction of missing or ablated jaw bone structure.

SUMMARY

The use of orthognathic surgery principles in manipulating edentulous arches, segments, and even small bone fragments to augment bone mass before implant placement appears to be sound practice. Although only recently done in the past decade to any great degree, the sandwich osteotomy and alveolar split grafting particularly aid in improving outcome in surgical efforts to recapture orthoalveolar form. In select cases, Le Fort procedures can be done for a total arch solution when atrophy is extreme, but most orthognathic surgery manipulations required are intra-arch segmental or intra-alveolar procedures that have the same power to transform an edentulous deformity as observed with orthognathic procedures done for dentate dentofacial deformities.

REFERENCES

1. Cheever DW. Naso-pharyngeal polypus, attached to the basilar process of occipital and body of the sphenoid bone successfully removed by a section,

displacement, and subsequent replacement and reunion of the superior maxillary bone. Boston Med Surg J 1867;8:162.

2. Trauner R, Obwegeser H. The surgical correction of mandibular prognathism and retrognathia with consideration of genioplasty. I. Surgical procedures to correct mandibular prognathism and reshaping of the chin. Oral Surg Oral Med Oral Pathol 1957;10(7):677–89.

3. Obwegeser HL. Surgical correction of small or retrodisplaced maxillae. The "dish-face" deformity. Plast Reconstr Surg 1969;43(4):351–65.

4. Bell WH. Revascularization and bone healing after anterior maxillary osteotomy: a study using adult rhesus monkeys. J Oral Surg 1969;27(4):249–55.

5. Bell WH, Levy BM. Revascularization and bone healing after anterior mandibular osteotomy. J Oral Surg 1970;28(3):196–203.

6. Olson RE, McMahon R, Winer H. Orthognathic surgery. Surg Clin North Am 1973; 53(1):253–76.

7. Kraut RA. Preprosthetic orthognathic surgery. Gen Dent 1984;32(3):250–4.

8. Bedhet N, Mercier J, Gordeeff A. Orthognathic surgery of the edentulous: a particular form of preprosthetic surgery. Actual Odontostomatol (Paris) 1989; 43(167):449–65 [in French].

9. Rosen PS, Forman D. The role of orthognathic surgery in the treatment of severe dentoalveolar extrusion. J Am Dent Assoc 1999;130(11):1619–22.

10. van der Mark EL, Bierenbroodspot F, Baas EM, et al. Reconstruction of an atrophic maxilla: comparison of two methods. Br J Oral Maxillofac Surg 2010. in press.

11. Sverzut CE, Trivellato AE, Sverzut AT, et al. Rehabilitation of severely resorbed edentulous mandible using the modified visor osteotomy technique. Braz Dent J 2009;20(5):419–23.

12. Jensen OT. Alveolar segmental "sandwich" osteotomies for posterior edentulous mandibular sites for dental implants. J Oral Maxillofac Surg 2006;64(3):471–5.

13. Jensen OT, Kuhlke L, Bedard JF, et al. Alveolar segmental sandwich osteotomy for anterior maxillary vertical augmentation prior to implant placement. J Oral Maxillofac Surg 2006;64(2):290–6.

14. González-García R, Monje F, Moreno C. Alveolar split osteotomy for the treatment of the severe narrow ridge maxillary atrophy: a modified technique. Int J Oral Maxillofac Surg 2011;40(1):57–64.

15. Scipioni A, Bruschi GB, Calesini G. The edentulous ridge expansion technique: a five-year study. Int J Periodontics Restorative Dent 1994;14(5):451–9.

16. Le B, Burstein J, Sedghizadeh PP. Cortical tenting grafting technique in the severely atrophic alveolar ridge for implant site preparation. Implant Dent 2008; 17(1):40–50.

17. Jensen OT, Bell W, Cottam J. Osteoperiosteal flaps and local osteotomies for alveolar reconstruction [review]. Oral Maxillofac Surg Clin North Am 2010;22(3): 331–46, vi.

18. Carvalho RS, Nelson D, Kelderman H, et al. Guided bone regeneration to repair an osseous defect. Am J Orthod Dentofacial Orthop 2003;123(4):455–67.

19. Jensen OT, Mogyoros R, Owen Z, et al. Island osteoperiosteal flap for alveolar bone reconstruction. J Oral Maxillofac Surg 2010;68(3):539–46.

20. Marchetti C, Trasarti S, Corinaldesi G, et al. Interpositional bone grafts in the posterior mandibular region: a report on six patients. Int J Periodontics Restorative Dent 2007;27(6):547–55.

21. Kahnberg KE, Vannas-Löfqvist L. Sinus lift procedure using a 2-stage surgical technique: I. Clinical and radiographic report up to 5 years. Int J Oral Maxillofac Implants 2008;23(5):876–84.

22. Papa F, Cortese A, Maltarello MC, et al. Outcome of 50 consecutive sinus lift operations. Br J Oral Maxillofac Surg 2005;43(4):309–13.
23. Bloomquist DS, Feldman GR. The posterior ilium as a donor site for maxillo-facial bone grafting. J Maxillofac Surg 1980;8(1):60–4.
24. Tonetti MS, Hämmerle CH, European Workshop on Periodontology Group C. Advances in bone augmentation to enable dental implant placement: consensus Report of the Sixth European Workshop on Periodontology. J Clin Periodontol 2008;35(8 Suppl):168–72.
25. Slavkin HC. Clinical dentistry in the 21st century. Compend Contin Educ Dent 1997;18(3):212–6, 218.
26. Schwartz Z, Somers A, Mellonig JT, et al. Addition of human recombinant bone morphogenetic protein-2 to inactive commercial human demineralized freeze-dried bone allograft makes an effective composite bone inductive implant material. J Periodontol 1998;69(12):1337–45.
27. Jensen OT, Leopardi A, Gallegos L. The case for bone graft reconstruction including sinus grafting and distraction osteogenesis for the atrophic edentulous maxilla. J Oral Maxillofac Surg 2004;62(11):1423–8.
28. Kroczek A, Park J, Birkholz T, et al. Effects of osteoinduction on bone regeneration in distraction: results of a pilot study. J Craniomaxillofac Surg 2010;38(5): 334–44.
29. Jensen OT, Kuhlke KL, Cottam J, et al. Maxillary alveolar split horseshoe osteotomy. In: Jensen OT, editor. The osteoperiosteal flap. Hanover Park (IL): Quintessence; 2010. p. 189–201.
30. Robiony M, Costa F. Sandwich osteotomy bone graft in the anterior maxilla. In: Jensen OT, editor. The osteoperiosteal flap. Hanover Park (IL): Quintessence; 2010. p. 131–41.
31. Jensen OT. Sandwich osteotomy combinedwith extraction socket bone graft. In: Jensen OT, editor. The osteoperiosteal flap. Hanover Park (IL): Quintessence; 2010. p. 143–53.
32. Fiorellini JP, Howell TH, Cochran D, et al. Randomized study evaluating recombinant human bone morphogenetic protein-2 for extraction socket augmentation. J Periodontol 2005;76(4):605–13.
33. Epker BN. Vascular considerations in orthognathic surgery. II. Maxillary osteotomies. Oral Surg Oral Med Oral Pathol 1984;57(5):473–8.
34. Enislidis G, Wittwer G, Ewers R. Preliminary report on a staged ridge splitting technique for implant placement in the mandible: a technical note. Int J Oral Maxillofac Implants 2006;21(3):445–9.
35. Araújo MG, Lindhe J. Dimensional ridge alterations following tooth extraction. An experimental study in the dog. J Clin Periodontol 2005;32(2):212–8.
36. Qahash M, Susin C, Polimeni G, et al. Bone healing dynamics at buccal peri-implant sites. Clin Oral Implants Res 2008;19(2):166–72.
37. Jensen OT, Mogyoros R, Alterman M, et al. Island osteoperiosteal flap. In: Jensen OT, editor. The osteoperiosteal flap. Hanover Park (IL): Quintessence; 2010. p. 101–14.
38. Jensen OT, Greer RO Jr, Johnson L, et al. Vertical guided bone-graft augmentation in a new canine mandibular model. Int J Oral Maxillofac Implants 1995;10(3): 335–44.
39. Herford AS, Boyne PJ. Reconstruction of mandibular continuity defects with bone morphogenetic protein-2 (rhBMP-2). J Oral Maxillofac Surg 2008;66(4): 616–24.

40. Boyne PJ. Application of bone morphogenetic proteins in the treatment of clinical oral and maxillofacial osseous defects. J Bone Joint Surg Am 2001;83(Suppl 1[Pt 2]): S146–50.
41. Urban IA, Jovanovic SA, Lozada JL. Vertical ridge augmentation using guided bone regeneration (GBR) in three clinical scenarios prior to implant placement: a retrospective study of 35 patients 12 to 72 months after loading. Int J Oral Maxillofac Implants 2009;24(3):502–10.
42. Llambés F, Silvestre FJ, Caffesse R. Vertical guided bone regeneration with bioabsorbable barriers. J Periodontol 2007;78(10):2036–42.
43. Romero-Olid Mde N, Vallencillo-Capilla M. A pilot study in the development of indeces for presiucting the clinical outcomes of oral bone grafts. Int J Oral Maxillofac Implants 2005;20:595–604.
44. de Carvalho PS, Vasconcellos LW, Pi J. Influence of bed preparation on the incorporation of autogenous bone grafts: a study in dogs. Int J Oral Maxillofac Implants 2000;15:565–70.
45. Jensen OT. Distraction osteogenesis and its use with dental implants. Dent Implantol Update 1999;10(5):33–6.
46. Gillot L, Noharet R, Cannas B. Guided surgery and presurgical prosthesis: preliminary results of 33 fully edentulous maxillae treated in accordance with the NobelGuide protocol. Clin Implant Dent Relat Res 2010;12(Suppl 1). e104–e13.
47. Jensen OT, Adams MW. The maxillary M-4: a technical and biomechanical note for all-on-4 management of severe maxillary atrophy—report of 3 cases. J Oral Maxillofac Surg 2009;67(8):1739–44 [erratum in: J Oral Maxillofac Surg 2009;67(11):2554].
48. Ferri J, Dujoncquoy JP, Carneiro JM, et al. Maxillary reconstruction to enable implant insertion: a retrospective study of 181 patients. Head Face Med 2008;4:31.
49. Sailer HF. A new method of inserting endosseous implants in totally atrophic maxillae. J Craniomaxillofac Surg 1989;17(7):299–305.
50. Collins TA, Brown GK, Johnson N, et al. Team management of atrophic edentulism with autogenous inlay, veneer, and split grafts and endosseous implants: case reports. Quintessence Int 1995;26(2):79–93.
51. Jensen OT, Cullum DR, Baer D. Marginal bone stability using 3 different flap approaches for alveolar split expansion for dental implants: a 1-year clinical study. J Oral Maxillofac Surg 2009;67(9):1921–30.
52. Nyström E, Nilson H, Gunne J, et al. Reconstruction of the atrophic maxilla with interpositional bone grafting/Le Fort I osteotomy and endosteal implants: a 11–16 year follow-up. Int J Oral Maxillofac Surg 2009;38(1):1–6.
53. Bell WH, Levy BM. Revascularization and bone healing after posterior maxillary osteotomy. J Oral Surg 1971;29(5):313–20.
54. Cho BC, Lee JH, Baik BS, et al. Distraction osteogenesis of free interpositional membranous bone: experimental design. J Craniofac Surg 1999;10(2):123–7.
55. Obradović O, Todorovic L, Vitanovic V. Anatomical considerations relevant to implant procedures in the mandible. Bull Group Int Rech Sci Stomatol Odontol 1995;38(1–2):39–44.
56. Pogrel MA, Dodson T, Tom W. Arteriographic assessment of patency of the inferior alveolar artery and its relevance to alveolar atrophy. J Oral Maxillofac Surg 1987;45(9):767–70.
57. Funaki K, Takahashi T, Yamuchi K. Horizontal alveolar ridge augmentation using distraction osteogenesis: comparison with a bone-splitting method in a dog model. Oral Surg Oral Med Oral Pathol Oral Radiol Endod 2009;107(3):350–8.

58. Laster Z, Rachmiel A, Jensen OT. Alveolar width distraction osteogenesis for early implant placement. J Oral Maxillofac Surg 2005;63(12):1724–30 [erratum in: J Oral Maxillofac Surg 2006;64(3):566].
59. Proffit WR, Turvey TA, Phillips C. The hierarchy of stability and predictability in orthognathic surgery with rigid fixation: an update and extension. Head Face Med 2007;3:21.

Craniofacial Implant Surgery

Douglas P. Sinn, DDS[a],*, Edmond Bedrossian, DDS[b],
Allison K. Vest, MBBS, MS, CCA[c]

KEYWORDS

- Cranial implants • Facial reconstruction
- Craniofacial congenital defects • Acquired facial defects

Reconstruction of acquired or congenitally absent facial structures such as ears, eyes, the nose, and other structures is a challenging task for the reconstructive surgeon. Often, inadequate soft tissue, cartilaginous structure, or osseous structure exists for a reconstruction that is both functional and aesthetic.

The use of external titanium cranial implants for prosthetic reconstruction in the head and neck region was developed from the pioneering work of Branemark, Briene, Adell Lindstrom, and other investigators in the late 1960s and early 1970s.[1–5] Because this technology emerged as a reliable reconstruction method for the maxillofacial/oral region, early work began regarding extraoral applications of the titanium osseointegrated implant. Initially, concerns regarding long-term stability and recurrent infection were vocalized by many investigators. Subsequently, however, work in the late 1970s and early 1980s by Tjellstrom, Albrektsson, Branemark, and Lindstrom revealed that the extraoral application of titanium implants for prosthetic reconstruction, bone-anchored conductive hearing aids, and other applications was a reliable technique.[6–12] Following the initial application of this technology for auricular reconstruction, other reconstructive procedures using osseointegrated retention such as orbital, nasal, and frontal prostheses have been evaluated in the literature.

PROSTHETIC RECONSTRUCTION

Most researchers agree that prosthetic reconstruction of the ear results in a cosmetically superior result when than that of autogenous reconstruction. This disparity does

This article was previously published in the May 2011 issue of *Oral and Maxillofacial Surgery Clinics of North America.*
[a] Division of Oral and Maxillofacial Surgery, Department of Surgery, UT Southwestern Medical School at Dallas, 5323 Harry Hines Boulevard, Dallas, TX 75390, USA
[b] Implant Training, Department of Oral and Maxillofacial Residency Training Program, Dugoni School of Dentistry, 2155 Webster Street, San Francisco, CA 94115, USA
[c] Medical Arts Prosthetics, LLC, 10501 North Central Expressway, Suite 314, Dallas, TX 75231, USA
* Corresponding author. 1752 North Broad Park Circle, Suite 100, Mansfield, TX 76063.
E-mail address: drsinn@afoms.com

dental.theclinics.com

not imply that traditional reconstructive techniques cannot achieve an excellent aesthetic result; however, the complex anatomy of structures such as the ears and nose can be extremely difficult to reconstruct and nearly impossible to replicate with traditional reconstructive surgery. Implant-retained prostheses offer an excellent reconstructive option that provides for excellent symmetry, color, and anatomic detail. Further, prosthetic reconstruction offers a rescue option for unacceptable or failed autogenous grafting procedures.[12–14]

Implant-retained prostheses offer several advantages over more traditional prosthetic techniques. Cranial implants provide secure attachment of the prosthesis that obviates the need for adhesives, double-sided tape, glasses, or other more traditional fixation methods, which may compromise prosthetic stability. Cranial implants enhance the patient's quality of life via improved self-image, greater activity level due to superior retention, and ease of prosthesis management. Traditional adhesives have several disadvantages such as discoloration of the prosthesis, skin reactions (especially in irradiated areas), and poor performance during activity or perspiration.[12,13,15] Another significant advantage of cranial implantation is that the technique avoids distortion of tissues inherent in traditional surgical reconstruction, which allows for superior tumor surveillance. It has been suggested, despite difficulties with osseointegration in irradiated bone, that cranial implants may have an advantage in the irradiated patient who has poor-quality soft tissues available for reconstruction.[16]

Several disadvantages to prosthetic reconstruction exist, including the necessity of prosthetic or implant maintenance because of normal wear and discoloration and depending on the level of the patient's activity. The prosthesis may be dislodged at inopportune times such as during social or athletic events, and some investigators have noted that some patients may have adverse psychological effects related to the prosthesis.[12–15]

AUTOGENOUS RECONSTRUCTION

The advantages of using autogenous tissue in head and neck reconstruction follow the generally accepted principles of reconstruction, that is, stable long-term reconstruction with living tissue with an intact blood supply. An inherent advantage with autogenous reconstruction is the potential to fight infection and heal.[14,15] In addition, the cartilaginous framework may have some growth potential in younger patients.[17] Traditional techniques allow for reconstruction of partial deformities (preserving local tissue), whereas prosthetic reconstruction is usually reserved for total loss of the structure and may actually require removal of local tissues to facilitate prosthetic rehabilitation. Traditional reconstruction may be a superior option for the poorly compliant patient as well. An added advantage is the elimination of prosthetic support and maintenance, which can be a significant expense to the patient.

The primary disadvantage of autogenous reconstruction is that the final result is often less than satisfactory to the surgeon, and the patient, in terms of aesthetic outcome.[18] In reference to auricular reconstruction, Wilkes noted, "the final reconstructed ear is acceptable aesthetically but less likely to exactly match the contralateral side when compared to a prosthetic ear."[14] Autogenous reconstruction generally requires multiple-staged procedures and may necessitate the use of tissue expansion, multiple grafts, or adjacent tissue transfers (such as a temporoparietal flap). Such procedures are technically more demanding and may increase the risk of surgical complications such as flap necrosis, nerve injury, alopecia, and infection. Greater surgical and donor site morbidities (ie, costochondral grafting) are further disadvantages to traditional reconstructive surgery. The time required for reconstruction is another issue to consider, with the average time for classic 4-stage reconstruction being around 9 to 18 months, with an additional 3 months if tissue expansion is required. For prosthetic reconstruction (in the nonirradiated patient) with cranial implants, only 3 to 5 months is needed.[14]

TEMPORAL IMPLANTS

In the case of temporal bone cranial implants for auricular reconstruction, an anteriorly or inferiorly based subperiosteal flap is the most preferred. Careful dissection to avoid perforation is necessary, especially in the previously operated patient or in the preoperatively irradiated region. The subcutaneous region of the flap is meticulously thinned in order to prevent soft tissue mobility around the implant. The presence of soft tissue mobility at the implant/soft tissue interface may lead to significant soft tissue reactions.[19] An appropriate (approximately ≥25 mm) amount of the flap width is maintained to ensure vascularity of the pedicle. Lundgren and colleagues[20] proposed the ideal positioning parameters and recommended placement approximately 18 mm from the external auditory canal at the 6-, 9-, and 12-o'clock positions for the right ear and at the 12-, 3-, and 6-o'clock positions for the left ear. The distance between implants should be approximately 11 mm (center to center). Generally, the authors have found these estimates to be accurate; however, local anatomic considerations often necessitate the placement of implants into nonideal locations. Prosthetic reconstruction should still be possible, provided the surgeon does not exceed the parameters outlined by the surgical guide. The implant-retaining magnets must be contained within the confines of the final prosthesis in order to achieve an optimal outcome. It is important to position the implants so that the final prosthetic ear is as symmetric as possible.

The complication rate is extremely low, although dural exposure may occur in some patients during the surgical procedure, which can be managed conservatively, usually healing uneventfully. In general, middle cranial fossa or sigmoid sinus exposure does not create a problem in most cases. Injury to aberrant anatomic variants of the intratemporal portion of the facial nerve is rare but should be considered when operating on younger patients or patients with craniofacial anomalies.[19,21,22]

ORBITAL IMPLANTS

Because of the osseous anatomy of the orbit, orbital implants must be placed radially within the orbital rim to provide adequate bone thickness for retention. Generally, implant placement within the lateral rim is recommended because of the increased thickness of the bone in this region. The authors have found the medial orbit to be problematic in most cases, secondary to lack of adequate bone and increased anatomic complexity due to the lacrimal fossa. Unfortunately, this means that the desired axial loading of the implants is impossible in this region, which is less favorable biomechanically than other craniofacial implant regions. Therefore, meticulous technique and consideration for staged bone grafting may be required for a successful implant-retained orbital prosthesis. Usually, 3 to 4 implants are placed in the lateral rim to provide adequate prosthetic stability. Further, the implants must be placed sufficiently within the orbit, slightly behind the rim, to allow adequate prosthetic thickness to provide camouflage for implant fixtures.

NASAL IMPLANTS

Implantation of the nasal region can be technically challenging because of the poor availability of quality bone. The more complex anatomy of the nasal cavity and the thin friable tissue in the area add to the difficulty of cranial implantation in this region. This difficulty is especially true for the irradiated patient. Implants are generally placed in a triangular arrangement, with 1 fixture placed superiorly (radix) and 2 placed in a lateral position to the frontal process of the maxilla. The implants must be placed slightly within the nasal cavity to engage adequate bone and, as in the case of the orbital reconstruction, provide for adequate prosthetic thickness.

SURGICAL TECHNIQUE

When considering the placement of maxillofacial implants in any type of maxillofacial defect, the fixtures should be placed with the planned prosthetic framework in mind. The angle of the implants should allow an emergence profile, allowing for a proper prosthetic design without interfering with the ideal sculpture of the prosthesis. Misplaced implants may cause poor aesthetic outcome. Proper spacing and angles of the implants are necessary to allow manipulation of the prosthetic components.

Computer-Guided Treatment Planning

The Maxillofacial Concept software allows collaboration between the surgeon, the maxillofacial prosthodontist, and/or the anaplastologist in treatment planning for the patient with maxillofacial defects. The 2-dimensional Digital Imaging and Communications in Medicine (DICOM) files of the patient are converted into a 3-dimensional (3D) format, allowing better visualization of the remaining osseous tissues by the surgical team. The patient's soft tissue can also be reformatted and superimposed onto the reconfigured 3D bone volume, showing the topography of the patient's remaining facial and intraoral architecture.

The maxillofacial prosthodontist and the anaplastologist can assess the thickness of the soft tissue and guide the surgical team in locating implants, abutments, and the prosthetic framework. By using the information provided by the Maxillofacial Concept software, the team can plan implant positions that best comply with surgical and the prosthetic principles. The surgical team can preoperatively position implants, evaluate angulation and the trajectory (**Fig. 1**), select final abutments (**Fig. 2**), and modify the treatment plan as needed until optimal implant positions for the support of the

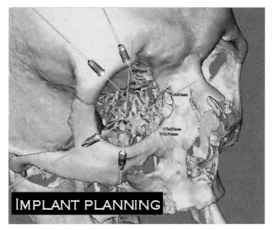

Fig. 1. The maxillofacial concept software allows the 3D active positioning of the implants during treatment planning.

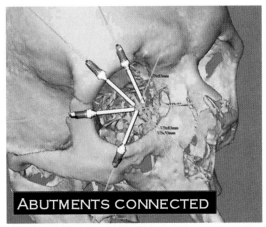

Fig. 2. Addition of abutments to the planned implant positions allows for better visualization of the trajectory of the implants.

maxillofacial prosthesis are obtained. The goal is to have a transparent transition line and aesthetic emergence profile. The final treatment plan is then taken to the operating room and the "virtual surgery" performed in the actual patient (**Fig. 3**).

Overlying soft tissues
Equal importance is given to the presence of healthy overlying and surrounding peri-implant soft tissues. Whether it is cutaneous or mucosal tissue, the clinicians must be aware of the thickness of the tissues to allow a maintainable environment around the prosthetic substructures. The management of the periabutment soft tissue is similar to intraoral management of soft tissue surrounding abutments. Thinning of flaps is usually necessary to allow a maintainable depth of soft tissue around the maxillofacial abutments.

Transition line
The transition line of the prosthesis with the patient's skin should be subtle and low profile for a lifelike appearance (**Fig. 4**). In any type of defect, the fixtures should be

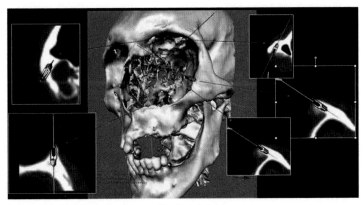

Fig. 3. Virtual surgery of a complex maxillofacial defect.

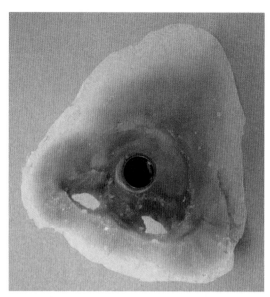

Fig. 4. Feathered margin of the prosthesis allows for a subtle transition line between the prosthesis and the patient's skin.

placed with the planned prosthetic framework in mind. The placement of the implants should allow for adequate emergence profile, allowing for proper bar design and/or magnet placement without interfering with the ideal sculpture of the prosthesis. Proper spacing and angles of the implants are also necessary to allow manipulation of the prosthetic screws by drivers that are needed during fabrication and delivery of the maxillofacial prosthesis.

Extraoral implants

Craniofacial implants can be regular platform implants. Extraoral implants used to date include machined surface, regular platform, 4.0-mm BrÅnemark implants. However, extraoral implants used for the BAHA (Cochlears Americas, Englewood, CA, USA) appliance or to support a prosthetic ear are not regular platform BrÅnemark implants. Implants used for the ear prosthesis are specially designed to support ear reconstruction or the BAHA appliance. Vistafix (Cochlears Americas, Englewood, CA, USA) implants, also developed by BrÅnemark (currently revised), are now the implants of choice for ear prosthetic stability and BAHA hearing aids **(Fig. 5)**. They are available in 3.0 and 4.0 mm lengths, with a 1.5-mm collar that is slightly submerged in the bone to increase the area of bone contact surface **(Fig. 6)**. Vistafix implants may be used for the ear, nose, and orbit.

Intraoral and intranasal implants

Intraoral and intranasal implants are also the machined surface regular platform implants or cranial implants available from Vistafix (Cochlear). If zygomatic bone is used for anchoring implants, several approaches were considered. For patients having had partial or total maxillectomies, regular platform implants were used in the remaining portion of the zygomatic body to allow for contralateral point stabilization of the prosthetic framework. If the maxillary residual arch is intact, the BrÅnemark zygomatic implant with the 45° angulated platform can also be used.

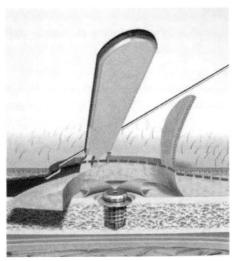

Fig. 5. Vistafix cranial implant for temporal bone with collar to increase surface area because the 3 and 4 mm lengths of the implant provide limited surface area.

Preparing the osteotomy

Most cases are treated in the operating room under general anesthesia. After sterile preparation and draping of the patient, lidocaine with epinephrine is administered to the surgical field to allow better control of hemostasis. Sharp dissection through the epithelium, the connective tissue, and the periosteum exposes the residual bony defect. The drilling sequence to prepare the osteotomy is the same as that for conventional intraoral implants. The surgeon has to judge clinically the quality of bone while preparing the osteotomy. When using cranial implants (Vistafix) the osteotomy can be completed with 1 specially designed drill that is either 3 or 4 mm in length and creates the collar osteotomy simultaneously (see **Fig. 6**).

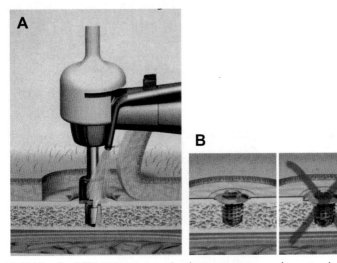

Fig. 6. (*A, B*) Vistafix drill bit that creates implant osteotomy and countersink for the collar simultaneously.

Orbital Defects

Placement of 2 to 3 implants is generally adequate for support of the substructure and the orbital prosthesis. The preferred site is the lateral supraorbital rim, if it has not been resected. However, implants may be placed in the residual periorbital bony rim. A special consideration in treatment planning of the orbital prosthesis is the available depth of the orbital defect. Inadequate orbital depths do not allow the tipping of the trajectory of the implant into the center of the orbit, resulting in inadequate space for the fabrication of the substructure and the orbital prosthesis. Virtual planning of the implants is performed, and the orbital depth is established intraoperatively by debulking the orbital contents. The implants are placed as planned at 35 N cm (**Fig. 7**). Immediate postoperative implant positioning must be done in conjunction with proposed virtual planning. Computer-guided treatment planning allows positioning of the implants in appropriate bony volume in concert with the proper trajectory for reconstruction of the maxillofacial prosthesis (**Fig. 8**). After exposure of the orbital rim, a round bur is used to identify the implant position (**Fig. 9**). On completion of the 2 mm osteotomy, a paralleling pin is placed to evaluate the trajectory (**Fig. 10**). The final osteotomy depth of 3 mm is followed by insertion of the implant. Most procedures follow a 1-stage protocol in which the temporary healing abutment is placed at the time of the implant surgery, with adaptation of the soft tissues (**Figs. 11** and **12**). Once the second implant is placed, the position of the actual surgery can be compared with the virtual surgery using the treatment planning software. Triple antibiotic ointment application and periimplant surface pressure dressings complete the surgical treatment. Osseointegration for 3 to 4 months is followed by fabrication of the substructure and the prosthetic device (**Figs. 13** and **14**).

Nasal Defects

Placement of the implants for supporting a nasal prosthesis is unique because access by the maxillofacial prosthodontist must be considered during treatment planning for

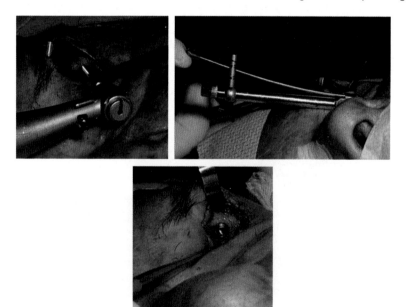

Fig. 7. The implants are placed with 35 N cm insertion torque.

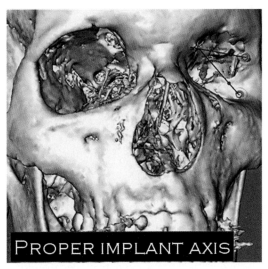

Fig. 8. Preoperative virtual planning of a 30-year-old man for implants to support an orbital prosthesis.

the position of the implants. The generally accessible bone volumes, which can support the implants, are in the premaxilla. Placing 2 implants through the nasal floor at positions corresponding with the dental positions No. 7 and No. 10 is recommended (**Fig. 15**). During treatment planning, especially in the fully dentate patient, consideration of vital structures, including the teeth and nasopalatine canals, is essential. The use of the maxillofacial planning software allows for visualization for avoiding vital structures (**Fig. 16**). Aesthetic considerations of the final prosthesis must also be considered. In cases in which oncological resection was not orchestrated with maxillofacial reconstruction, the excess soft tissue can hinder an aesthetic prosthetic outcome (**Fig. 17**).

Following virtual treatment planning, 2 implants are placed with implant platforms tilted outward to allow easy access by the maxillofacial prosthodontist. The 1-stage surgical protocol is followed. However, it is prudent to place the final abutment at the time of surgery. Placement of the final abutment and impression coping at the time of surgery are done in conjunction with placement of a triple antibiotic pressure

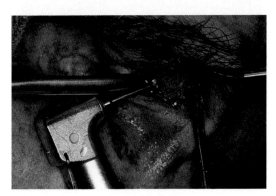

Fig. 9. To initiate the osteotomy, a round bur is used.

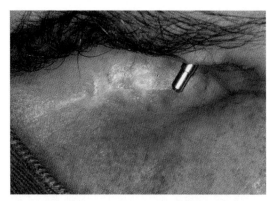

Fig. 10. A paralleling pin demonstrates the trajectory of the 2 mm osteotomy.

dressing, which allows for adaptation of the nasal mucosa to the nasal floor. It is not advisable to place a third implant in the nasal bone because the nasal prosthesis is adequately retained with 2 implants. There is no biomechanical advantage to placing a third implant, and the emergence profile of a third implant generally interferes with natural contours of the prosthetic nasal bridge. After a 3- to 4-month osseointegration period, a magnet-retained prosthesis is fabricated (**Fig. 18**).

Healing Period

A 2-stage surgical protocol may be used per the surgical team's preference. For a 2-stage approach, after installation of the implants, cover screws are placed and the implants submerged. Exposure of the implants is done later.

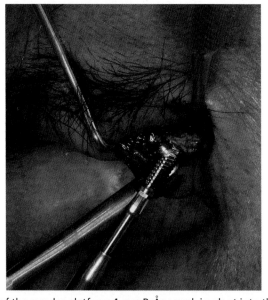

Fig. 11. Insertion of the regular platform 4-mm BrÅnemark implant into the osteotomy site.

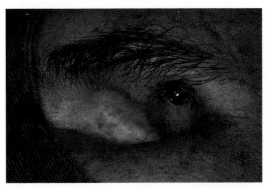

Fig. 12. Placement of a healing abutment completes the 1-stage protocol.

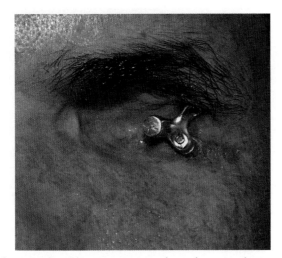

Fig. 13. Metal framework with a magnet used as the retentive component for the prosthesis.

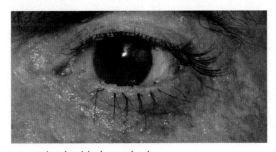

Fig. 14. Final magnet-retained orbital prosthesis.

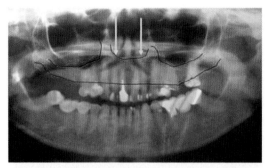

Fig. 15. Implants to retain a nasal prosthesis is placed through the nasal floor (*arrows*) in proximity to teeth Nos. 7 and 10.

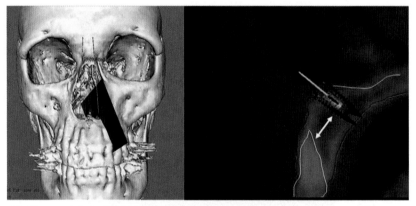

Fig. 16. The nasal floor, the hard palate, and the position of the existing teeth are readily visualized during the virtual planning. A safe distance is maintained between the vital teeth and the implant.

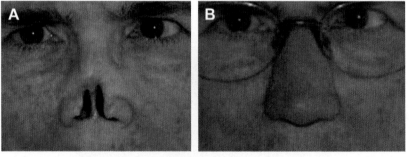

Fig. 17. (*A, B*) Inadequate resection and site preparation result in an unaesthetic transition line between the prosthesis and the patient's skin.

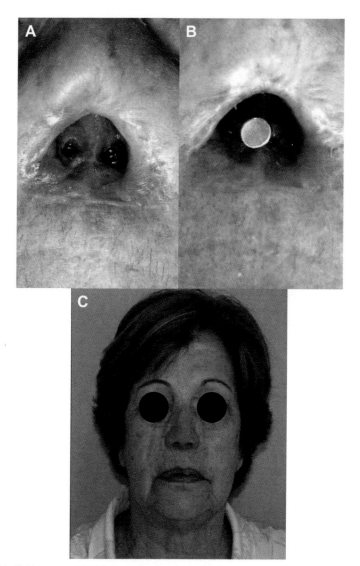

Fig. 18. (A–C) Abutment level impression is taken after osseointegration of the implants followed by fabrication of the superstructure and the final magnet-retained nasal prosthesis.

SOFT TISSUE REACTIONS AND INFECTIONS

The rate of soft tissue reactions around percutaneous implants has been reported to be between 3% and 60%, with significant variation reported depending on the stated definitions used to define a reaction.[23,24] Most investigators have noted soft tissue reactions in around 3% to 7% of percutaneous implants, with most of the reactions being mild erythema or irritation.[16,25] In a total of 2624 postoperative implant observations in 309 cranial implants (follow-up from 1–12 years), Westin and colleagues[19] reported a 3% incidence of significant skin reactions. Abu-Serriah and colleagues[26] found soft tissue infection to be the most common complication in a group of 150 cranial implants. They also observed a decreased infection incidence after the first 2 years of service in the temporal region. However, implants in the orbital and nasal regions exhibited a constant rate of soft tissue complications over time.

RADIATION AND CRANIAL IMPLANTATION

When using cranial implants for reconstruction of oncological defects of the facial skeleton, placement of implants into irradiated bone is inevitable. As with all irradiated tissues, soft tissue fibrosis coupled with the loss of the microvasculature occurs in the recipient bed. The resulting decreased oxygen tension has a negative effect on the ability to place titanium implants and obtain successful integration. Most investigators report significantly increased failure rates (ranging from 17%–42%) for cranial implants placed into irradiated bone.[16,21,27–30] When examining 81 cranial implants, Jacobsson and colleagues[25] described a success rate of 62.7% (vs 92.1% in nonirradiated bone). Implants that were lost in irradiated bone when placed after a 12-month period were generally successful. The orbit is an especially difficult location to achieve implant integration after radiation therapy.[31,32] In a group of 24 orbital implants, Roumanas and colleagues[22] observed a high rate of loss in the irradiated orbit and reported a 100% complication rate, with complications including failure to osseointegrate, late failure, tissue inflammation, and soft tissue recession. Successful implantation of the orbit is significantly more difficult to accomplish in the irradiated patient, with most studies reporting success rates in the range of 50% to 66%.[22,25,27] Despite the adverse effect of radiation regarding cranial implant osseointegration, the risk of craniofacial osteoradionecrosis is low and seldom observed.[16,22,27,31] The timing of implant placement at the conclusion of radiation therapy remains controversial with most researchers recommending a delay of 6 to 19 months before implant placement.[22,26,27]

The use of hyperbaric oxygen (HBO) has been advocated by multiple studies in the literature to improve integration rates and optimize soft tissue healing when placing cranial implants into irradiated bone.[16,26,27] When examining 125 irradiated cranial implants, Granstrom and colleagues[27] noted that 38.4% of irradiated implants were lost in the irradiated group versus 17% in the nonirradiated group. Of the irradiated implants, 45 received preoperative HBO therapy, and no implants were lost in this group. It was concluded that HBO was extremely beneficial in the irradiated field before the placement of cranial implants. In reference to the proposed soft tissue benefits of HBO, no statistical difference in local skin reactions was observed between patients who received HBO therapy and those who did not.

PROSTHETIC CONSIDERATIONS

A stable and consistent prosthetic attachment is crucial to the successful rehabilitation of the patient who underwent maxillofacial surgery. For the anaplastologist or practitioner who is designing and fabricating prostheses, implementing cranial implants can significantly help meet the needs of the patient. Anaplastology is commonly defined as the application of prosthetic materials for reconstruction of an absent, disfigured, or missing body part (from the Greek *ana* meaning again, and *plastos* meaning something made or formed). "The anaplastologist is charged with the formidable task of restoring the delicate beauty of the human ear."[33] This task is assigned and applied to all facial prosthetic reconstructions.

PREOPERATIVE PLANNING

Preoperative appointments with the anaplastologist are considered an integral part of the treatment planning process for patients requiring prosthetic reconstruction.[34] At the initial consultation, before and after photos of previous cases can be shown to help the patient visualize possible results and treatment options. The anaplastologist can effectively plan to achieve the highest level of realism and symmetry attainable under the given circumstances. When possible, presurgical impressions capturing natural anatomy before planned resections or tumor excision are helpful. This record of the patient's own facial features can help to establish a prosthetic design that the patient will ultimately recognize and relate. Discussion of all retention types should be initiated at this stage, with the advantages of each clearly explained.

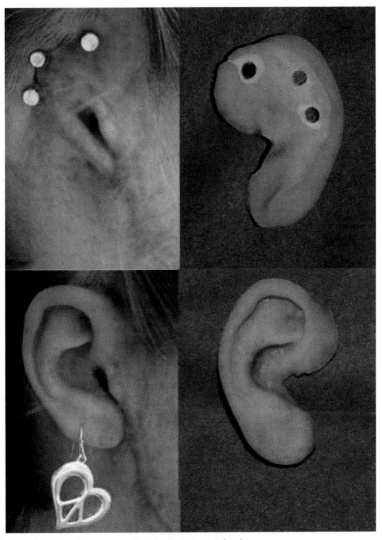

Fig. 19. The freestanding magnetic attachment method.

Options with Cranial Implant Surgery

An implant-retained prosthesis provides a secure and consistent method of attachment. The mechanical connection between the patient and the prosthesis can alleviate psychological concerns that the prosthesis will become loose or dislodge at any time.[35] It also ensures exact positioning without the need of a mirror or care giver. In addition, the life span of an implant-retained prosthesis is typically longer than that requiring adhesive because of the less wear and tear associated with the adhesive removal process.

When the surgically placed implant-retained type is chosen, the bar and clip versus magnetic attachment option should be decided presurgically (**Figs. 19** and **20**). This decision will determine how many exposed implants are needed. Experience has shown that the gold bar arrangement proves more difficult for many patients to clean

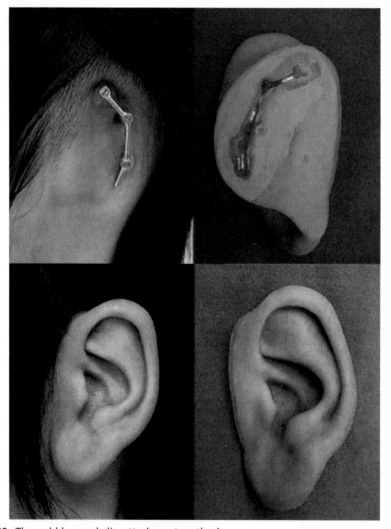

Fig. 20. The gold bar and clip attachment method.

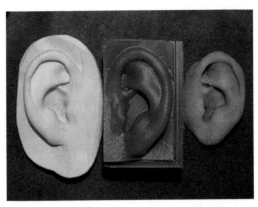

Fig. 21. Patient cast, prototyped model, and the final prosthesis, respectively.

than the freestanding abutments for magnetic attachment. The magnetic attachment requires little manual dexterity. The recently developed Maxi O-ring Magnet by MagnaCap System, Technovent Ltd, Newport, South Wales, UK, "provides far superior retention to that of conventional magnets."[36] In the authors' experience, using only 1 of these O-ring magnets in a prosthesis meets or surpasses the retention of a bar and clip design.

Auricular Considerations

Advancements in 3D technology, such as scanning and milling machines, provide for accurate reproduction of contralateral auricular forms. Using such devices helps the practitioner accurately and quickly achieve a certain level of symmetry (**Fig. 21**). The

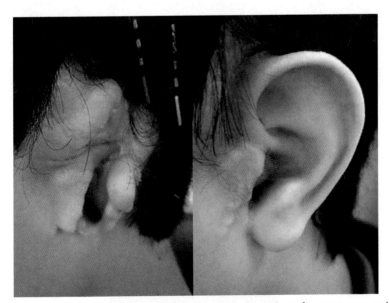

Fig. 22. Modification of cartilaginous tissue for the construction of a neotragus and prosthetic reconstruction.

patient's existing auricular cast is scanned, digitally mirror imaged, and milled in 3D. This shape gives the anaplastologist a reliable reference to design the final auricular prosthesis.

In congenital cases, there are often several options to consider. Cartilaginous remnants from failed autogenous reconstructions can be retained or sculpted and repositioned for the construction of a neotragus. The presence of a tragus allows the anterior prosthetic margins to be elegantly concealed behind this anatomic feature (**Fig. 22**). Symmetric and well-positioned microtic tissue can remain underneath an implant-retained auricular prosthesis. Microtic tissue compromising the aesthetic outcome should be removed at the time of implant placement. However, this step should be clearly discussed with the patient before surgery, thus allowing plenty of time for decision making. It is not uncommon for the patient to feel emotionally attached to his/her microtic remnant.

TEMPLATES

Implants should be placed in an area of the prosthesis that is thick enough to contain and naturally disguise retentive hardware. Designing a prototype prosthesis before surgery determines areas of thickness and other important features. The prototype

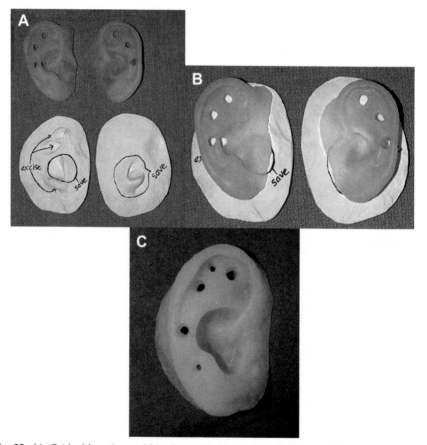

Fig. 23. (*A–C*) Ideal locations within the antihelix portion of the surgical template.

can then be used in the construction of the surgical template. The template should designate preferred implant locations (**Fig. 23**A, C) and other optional sites in case favored locations are not acceptable due to poor bone quality. Templates should conform passively to the surgical site during surgery. Nearby anatomic features should be built into the template design to ensure proper placement. Various materials, such as acrylic or silicone, are used in template fabrication.

Auricular Templates

The basic reference mark in locating potential auricular implant sites is the middle of the external auditory canal. Using this landmark, the ideal location is found to be approximately 20 mm from the center of the external auditory meatus. Using these locations within the template should allow for retentive hardware to be concealed in the antihelix portion of the prosthesis (see **Fig. 23**).

CONSTRUCTION OF THE PROSTHESIS

The final visual prosthetic result depends on achieving a delicate balance of many factors during all stages of construction. Fabrication begins with capturing an accurate impression. Soft tissue movement, areas of sensitivity, and hair surrounding the site should be taken into account.

An accurate impression material must be used to precisely register the abutments and record soft tissue. Applying 2 layers of polyvinyl siloxane material provides the required exactness. A thin light-bodied layer is applied followed by a heavy-bodied material to stabilize the impression hardware (**Fig. 24**). For magnetic attachments (see **Fig. 24**), the transfer magnet remains within the impression and is used for registering the laboratory analogue abutments within the cast. The cast obtained from this captured impression serves as the master cast on which the definitive prosthesis is

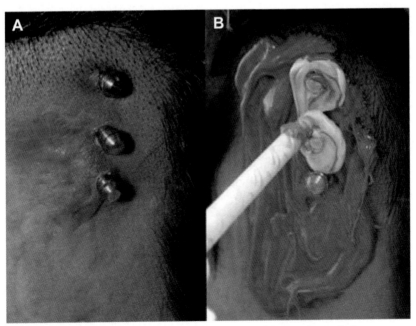

Fig. 24. (*A*) Transfer magnets in location. (*B*) Two-layered impression technique.

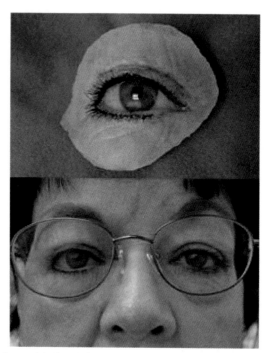

Fig. 25. Margins of an orbital prosthesis disguised behind the patient's frames.

built. Input and feedback from the patient should be especially encouraged during this stage. A prototype form should be tried on and examined by both the patient and the anaplastologist. The boundary of an orbital prosthesis can be effectively disguised behind the edges of the patient's glasses (**Fig. 25**).

Color and Tinting of the Prosthesis

Creating realistic skin colors in silicone requires selecting a combination of colorant that mimics the absorption and transmission of human skin.[37] To achieve a high level of realism, several factors must be taken into consideration: opacity/translucency, hue (color), value (too dark or too light), and chroma (intensity).[33] Various lighting conditions can alter any of these aspects of color.

The final result should be undetected at a normal conversational distance and should prevent the patient from having his/her condition recognized in social situations. This result transforms the patient's self-esteem and overall presentation. Symmetry, organic form, and attention to color detail contribute to the patient's acceptance of the prosthetic silicone feature.

SUMMARY

Extraoral cranial implant-retained prosthetic reconstructions have been proved to be highly successful. Replacement of the eyes, ears, nose, and larger areas including combined midface defects, which frequently have no other option available, has been done successfully. Burn patients and those with congenital defects are good candidates for this type of reconstruction, especially after autogenous attempts have failed. Cranial implant prosthetic reconstruction should be considered as a viable option for difficult craniofacial defects.

REFERENCES

1. Branemark PI, Adell R, Breine U, et al. Intra-osseous anchorage of dental prosthesis. I. Experimental studies. Scand J Plast Reconstr Surg 1969;3:81–100.
2. Adell R, Hansson BO, Branemark PI, et al. Intra-osseous anchorage of dental prosthesis. II. Review of clinical approaches. Scand J Plast Reconstr Surg 1970;4:19–34.
3. Branemark PI, Breine U, Hallen O, et al. Repair of defects in mandible. Scand J Plast Reconstr Surg 1970;4:100–8.
4. Branemark PI, Breine U, Adell R, et al. Experimentella studier av intraosseal forankring av dentala proteser. Rsbok/Goteborgs Tandlakare-Sallskaps 1970;9–25 [in Swedish].
5. Branemark PI, Adell R, Hansson BO. Kakrekonstruktion och benforankrand bettersattning. Tandlakartidningen 1971;63:486–97 [in Swedish].
6. Tjellstrom A, Hakansson B, Lindstrom J, et al. Analysis of the mechanical impedance of bone-anchored hearing aids. Acta Otolaryngol 1980;89:85–92.
7. Tjellstrom A, Lindstrom J, Nylen O, et al. The bone-anchored auricular episthesis. Laryngoscope 1981;91:811–915.
8. Albrektsson T, Branemark PI, Hansson HA, et al. Osseointegrated titanium implants. Requirements for ensuring a long-lasting direct bone-to-implant anchorage in man. Acta Orthop Scand 1981;52:155–70.
9. Tjellstrom A, Lindstrom J, Hallen O, et al. Osseointegrated titanium implants in the temporal bone. A clinical study on bone-anchored hearing aids. Am J Otol 1981; 2:304–10.
10. Branemark PI, Albrektsson T. Titanium implants permanently penetrating human skin. Scand J Plast Reconstr Surg 1982;16:17–21.
11. Tjellstrom A, Lindstrom J, Nylen O, et al. Directly bone-anchored implants for fixation of aural episthesis. Biomaterials 1983;4:55–7.
12. Tjellstrom A, Rosenhall U, Lindstrom J, et al. Five year experience with skin-penetrating bone-anchored implants in the temporal bone. Acta Otolaryngol 1983;95:568–75.
13. Tjellstrom A, Yontichev E, Lindstrom J, et al. Five years experience with bone-anchored auricular prosthesis. Otolaryngol Head Neck Surg 1985;93:366–72.
14. Wilkes GH, Wolfaardt J. Osseointegrated alloplastic versus autogenous ear reconstruction: criteria for treatment selection. Plast Reconstr Surg 1994;93: 967–79.
15. Wolfaardt JF, Tam V, Faulkner M, et al. Mechanical behavior of three maxillofacial prosthetic adhesive systems: a pilot project. J Prosthet Dent 1992;68:943.
16. Granstrom G, Tjellstrom A, Branemark P, et al. Bone-anchored reconstruction of the irradiated head and neck cancer patient. Otolaryngol Head Neck Surg 1993; 108:334–43.
17. Thomson HG, Winslow J. Microtia reconstruction: does the cartilage framework grow? Plast Reconstr Surg 1989;84:908.
18. Brent B. Personal approach to total auricular construction. Clin Plast Surg 1981;8: 211–21.
19. Westin T, Tjellstrom A, Hammerlid E, et al. Long-term study of quality and safety of osseointegration for the retention of auricular prostheses. Otolaryngol Head Neck Surg 1999;121:133–43.

20. Lundgren S, Moy PK, Beurmer J, et al. Surgical considerations for endosseous implants in the craniofacial region: a 3-year report. Int J Oral Maxillofac Surg 1993;22:272–7.
21. Wolfaardt J, Wilkes G, Parel S, et al. Craniofacial osseointegration: the Canadian experience. Int J Oral Maxillofac Implants 1993;8:197–204.
22. Roumanas E, Nishimura R, Beumer J, et al. Craniofacial defect and osseointegrated implants: six-year follow-up report on the success rates of craniofacial implants at UCLA. Int J Oral Maxillofac Implants 1994;9:579–85.
23. Abu-Serriah MM, McGowan DA, Moos KF, et al. Outcome of extraoral craniofacial endosseous implants. Br J Oral Maxillofac Surg 2001;39:269–75.
24. Holgers KM, Tjellstrom A. Soft tissue reaction around percutaneous implants: a clinical study on skin-penetrating titanium implants used for bone-anchored auricular prostheses. Int J Oral Maxillofac Implants 1987;2:35–8.
25. Jacobsson M, Tjellstrom A, Fine L, et al. A retrospective study of osseointegrated skin-penetrating titanium fixtures used for retaining facial prostheses. Int J Oral Maxillofac Implants 1992;75:523–8.
26. Abu-Serriah MM, McGowan DA, Moos KF, et al. Extraoral craniofacial endosseous implants and radiotherapy. Int J Oral Maxillofac Surg 2003;32:585–92.
27. Granstrom G, Bergstrom K, Tjellstrom A, et al. A detailed analysis of titanium implants 1994;653–62.
28. Scheon PJ, Raghoebar GM, Reinstema H, et al. Treatment outcome of bone-anchored craniofacial prostheses after tumor surgery. Cancer 2001;92(12): 3045–50.
29. Granstrom G, Jacobsson M, Tjellstrom A. Titanium implants in irradiated tissue: benefits from hyperbaric oxygen. Int J Oral Maxillofac Implants 1992;7:15–25.
30. Jacobsson M, Tjellstrom A, Thomsen P, et al. Integration of titanium implant in irradiated bone: histologic and clinical study. Ann Otol Rhinol Laryngol 1988;97:337–40.
31. Parel SM, Tjellstrom A. The United States and Swedish experience with osseointegration and facial prosthesis. Int J Oral Maxillofac Implants 1991;6:75–9.
32. Gion GG. Surgical versus prosthetic reconstruction of microtia. The case for prosthetic reconstruction. J Oral Maxillofac Surg 2006;64:1639–54.
33. Hemar P, Reidinger-Keller AM. Optimal surgical procedures following tumor resection for successful prosthetic rehabilitation by means of osseointegrated craniofacial implants. Int J Anaplast 2009;3:17–24.
34. Schaaf NG, Kielich M. Implant-retained facial prostheses. In: McKinstry RE, editor. Fundamental of facial prosthetics. Arlington (VA): ABI Professional Publications; 1995. p. 169–79.
35. Thomas KF. Prosthetic rehabilitation. London: Quintessence Publishing; 1994. 21. p. 169–93.
36. Vistafix® treatment guide. Engelwood (CO): Cochlear Americas; 2007. p. 17.
37. Tanner P. The use of light remittance measurements to determine intrinsic pigment concentrations in designing a realistic auricular prosthesis. Int J Anaplast 2008;2:7–14.

FURTHER READINGS

Belus JF, Kaplanski P, Blanc JL, et al. Orbito-maxillo-facial rehabilitation with osteointegrated prostheses. Ann Otolaryngol Chir Cervicofac 1996;113(7–8):397–407 [in French].
Cervelli V, Bottini DJ, Arpino A, et al. Orbital reconstruction: bone-anchored implants. J Craniofac Surg 2006;17(5):848–53.

Miles BA, Sinn DP, Gion GG. Experience with cranial implant-based prosthetic reconstruction. J Craniofac Surg 2006;17(5):889–97.

Roumanas ED, Chang TL, Beumer J. Use of osseointegrated implants in the restoration of head and neck defects. J Calif Dent Assoc 2006;34(9):711–8.

Schaaf NG. Maxillofacial prosthetics in the head and neck cancer patient. Cancer 1984;54(Suppl 11):2682–90.

Tolman DE, Tjellstrom A, Woods JE. Reconstructing the human face by using the tissue-integrated prosthesis. Mayo Clin Proc 1998;73(12):1171–5.

Van Doorne JM. Extra-oral prosthetics; past and present. J Invest Surg 1994;7(4): 267–74.

Dental Implants in Oral Cancer Reconstruction

D. David Kim, DMD, MD*, G.E. Ghali, DDS, MD

KEYWORDS

- Implants • Reconstruction • Jaw • Mandible
- Maxilla • Oral cancer

Endosseous implants have revolutionized dental prosthetic rehabilitation, providing a reliable, stable, and aesthetic option for dental reconstruction. Dental implants have similarly improved the functionality of reconstructions following cancer surgery. The use of dental implants in oral cancer reconstruction can be divided into 2 categories. First, for retention of a prosthetic device, for example, palatal obturator, used as the primary means of maxillary reconstruction. Second, for dental rehabilitation after bony reconstruction of the jaws. This article discusses these different uses of endosseous implants in patients with head and neck cancer.

IMPLANTS FOR MAXILLARY OBTURATORS

For more than a hundred years, use of the palatal obturator has been the principal mode of reconstruction of the maxilla after extirpative surgery and is still considered by many to be the gold standard in maxillary reconstruction. Depending on the nature of the defect (size, vertical extent of maxillary resection, degree of soft tissue loss, involvement of soft palate) and the status of the patient's dentition, the conventional obturator can function quite well as a means of restoring the dentition and separating the oral and nasal cavities (**Fig. 1**). However, many disadvantages of tissue- and tooth-borne devices are apparent.

In the partially dentate patient, the obturator is designed to function much like a removable partial denture, with support provided by the remaining palatal bone, the obturated cavity, and the remaining dentition. This situation may lead to

This article was previously published in the May 2011 issue of *Oral and Maxillofacial Surgery Clinics of North America*.

The authors have nothing to disclose.

Department of Oral and Maxillofacial Surgery, Head and Neck Surgery, Louisiana State University Health Sciences Center Shreveport, 1501 Kings Highway, Administration Building, Shreveport, LA 71103, USA

* Corresponding author.

E-mail address: dkim1@lsuhsc.edu

Dent Clin N Am 55 (2011) 871–882

doi:10.1016/j.cden.2011.07.013

0011-8532/11/$ – see front matter © 2011 Elsevier Inc. All rights reserved.

dental.theclinics.com

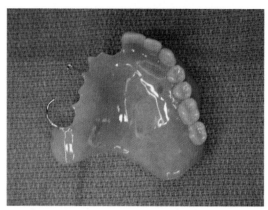

Fig. 1. Traditional maxillary obturator with retention clasps on remaining dentition.

unfavorable forces on the remaining dentition, compromising these teeth over time. In the edentulous patient, only the remaining hard palate, the maxillary alveolus, and the obturated cavity are available for support. In more extensive resections, there may be no maxillary bone present to provide obturator support, and therefore, very few options are available for conventional obturator use.

Similarly, retention of these prostheses can also be problematic. In the absence of the dentition, soft tissue retention at the interface of the buccal mucosa and the obturated cavity has been considered a primary retention principle in the fabrication of these devices. These devices have marginal levels of retention and are commonly a source of annoyance from constant irritation caused by the mobility of the prostheses. These factors also lead to a large bulk of material that can make the appliance difficult to handle and relatively heavy.

Endosseous and zygomatic implants can improve a patient's ability to wear these obturators by improving prosthetic stability and retention. In the edentulous patient, use of multiple endosseous implants in the residual alveolar bone can provide a platform for the fabrication of a retention bar that supports the overlying obturator prosthesis. Depending on the size and location of the defect, the forces placed on these implants can be unfavorable and can lead to eventual implant loss in a fashion similar to obturators supported by natural teeth in the partially edentulous patient. Placement of endosseous implants into the remaining bone surrounding the maxillary defect (pterygoid plates, zygoma, residual maxilla) (**Fig. 2**) has been advocated to avoid these

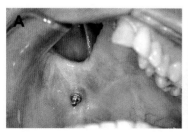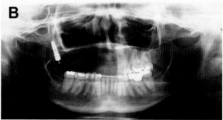

Fig. 2. (*A*) Traditional endosseous implant placed in the pterygoid plates to aid obturator stability in a patient who underwent right hemimaxillectomy. (*B*) Radiograph of the same patient.

unfavorable forces.[1] However, these implants have poor osteointegration potential and are difficult to restore and maintain.

Although the zygomatic implant was initially intended for aiding in the prosthetic rehabilitation of the atrophic maxillary alveolus,[2] it has been adapted often in combination with traditional endosseous implants for maxillary obturator support and retention.[3,4] Some of the limitations of implant placement in the bone surrounding the maxillectomy defect are mitigated by the use of these specialized implants, in that they are able to engage more distant bone. Very little literature exists on the use of zygomatic implants for this indication, and little is known about the long-term implications of these devices in maxillary reconstruction, but their use seems to be a reliable and effective adjunct to traditional implants for prosthesis support (**Fig. 3**). In a series by Schmidt and colleagues,[3] 21% of zygomatic implants failed at the time of stage II implant surgery. This relatively high implant failure rate was attributed to the use of radiation either before or after implant placement. Another case series reporting on a mixed group of patients receiving zygomatic implants for maxillectomies as well as traumatic injuries, severely atrophic maxillas, cleft lip, and cleft palate reported an overall failure rate of 5.9%.[5]

IMPLANTS IN RECONSTRUCTED JAWS

The reconstructive surgeon has several options for bony reconstruction of the maxilla or mandible. The specifics of different bone graft harvest sites or free flap donor sites are beyond the scope of this article, but the characteristics of some of these options as they pertain to implant reconstructions are worthy of mention. Regardless of the technique used for jaw reconstruction, the surgeon should consider the goal of full dental rehabilitation as the ultimate end point of the reconstruction.

Advancements in reconstructive surgery have taken cancer reconstruction from a high-risk afterthought of cancer treatment to a reliable and expected component

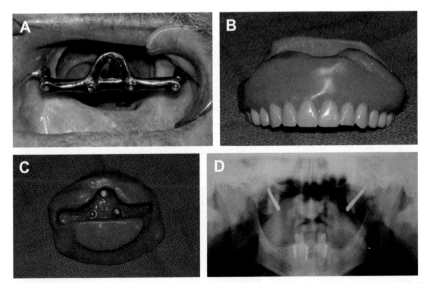

Fig. 3. (*A*) Patient who underwent near-total maxillectomy after resection for fungal infection with 2 zygomatic implants supporting a bar-retained obturator prosthesis. (*B, C*) Obturator designed to engage framework to aid in support and retention. (*D*) Radiograph of the same patient.

of cancer surgery. The use of regional flaps and free tissue transfer has allowed for more complex reconstructions and improved functional outcomes. Similarly, the necessity for dental reconstruction has followed with these advancements, and in many cases, it is no longer satisfactory to have a successful cancer ablation and an edentulous reconstructed jaw.

The time-honored gold standard in jaw reconstruction is the free iliac crest bone graft. Bone harvested from the anterior or posterior iliac crest is placed in a mandibular defect as a block or a corticocancellous graft, or a combination of the 2 (**Fig. 4**). Because of the nonvascular nature of these grafts, this procedure is generally performed as a secondary operation many months after the initial cancer ablation to avoid the high incidence of graft loss and infection when performed primarily. This type of mandible reconstruction is most suited for relatively short defects of the lateral mandible that do not cross the midline and is a highly effective technique for reconstruction in benign tumor resections such as ameloblastomas. The usefulness of this type of reconstruction is somewhat decreased in cancer reconstruction because many patients require postoperative radiation treatment that can inhibit bone graft healing and consolidation. Preoperative and postoperative hyperbaric oxygen (HBO) therapy and the use of regional flaps to provide vascularized tissue to the area have been advocated by some investigators to improve the vascular quality of the wound bed and graft healing.[6] Although useful in selected cases, the emergence of microvascular free tissue transfer has largely supplanted these techniques.

Composite microvascular tissue transfer has revolutionized cancer reconstruction, in that bone and soft tissue can be transferred from a distant site in the same operative encounter as the ablative surgery and, in most instances, from a single donor site. The literature is replete with various donor sites advocated for use in maxillary and mandibular reconstruction, including the ilium, fibula, scapula, radius, rib, and metatarsal. Each donor site has its own advantages and disadvantages, and an ideal replacement for maxillary or mandibular bone and intraoral soft tissue does not exist yet. However, of the donor sites currently available for jaw reconstruction, the ilium and fibula have emerged as the most desirable. Of these 2 sites, the fibula has numerous advantages over the ilium, with few drawbacks.

The iliac crest bone can be harvested as a bone-only, an osteocutaneous, or a myo-osteocutaneous (internal oblique) flap, based on the deep circumflex iliac artery (DCIA) and the accompanying deep circumflex iliac vein (DCIV). This flap's greatest advantage is the bone volume available for transfer, which is more than suitable for implant placement. Although the volume of the bone is good, the length of the bone available is somewhat limited, and the volume of soft tissue that must be included with this flap can be bulky (**Fig. 5**). The DCIA and DCIV provide a fair length of pedicle for mandible reconstruction, but their use in the maxilla usually requires vein grafts. Finally,

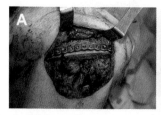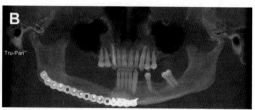

Fig. 4. (*A*) Secondary reconstruction of lateral mandibular defect with anterior iliac crest bone graft using a cortical block and cancellous marrow. (*B*) Radiograph of the consolidated bone graft in the same patient.

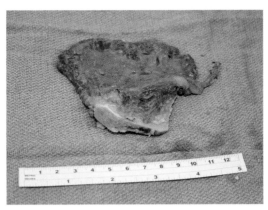

Fig. 5. Iliac crest flap with internal oblique muscle harvested. Note the relatively short pedicle length.

harvesting of the DCIA flap requires disruption of the anterior abdominal wall and upper leg muscle attachments, leading to hernias and gait disturbances, respectively. Collectively, these drawbacks have somewhat overshadowed this flap's significant bone volume advantage over the fibula and has affected its acceptance as a suitable donor site for jaw reconstruction. Accordingly, implantation into iliac crest grafts has not been reported much, and very little literature is available for review.

The fibula can also be harvested as a bone-only, an osteoseptocutaneous, or a myo-osteocutaneous flap (soleus or flexor hallucis longus). The fibula flap was introduced for use in mandible reconstruction in 1989 by Hidalgo[7] and has been the first choice for jaw reconstruction for many reconstructive surgeons. The fibula flap is popular for several reasons, including the ease of harvest, ability to work in 2 teams, availability of a long bony segment for harvest, low morbidity, and good pedicle length and caliber of vessels. Its disadvantages are few, but critics have argued that the bone is of insufficient height, has an inflexible skin paddle, and has the possibility of potential vascular compromise to the foot.

Much of the criticism regarding the effectiveness of the fibula in mandible reconstruction is aimed at its lack of vertical height. On average, the fibula's height is between 13 and 15 mm and is very close to that of an edentulous mandible (**Fig. 6**), but the fibula certainly lacks the height of a dentate mandible (**Fig. 7**). Various

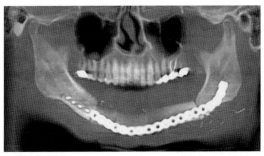

Fig. 6. Radiograph of fibula flap reconstruction of anterior mandible. The height of the fibula closely approximates the edentulous posterior right mandible.

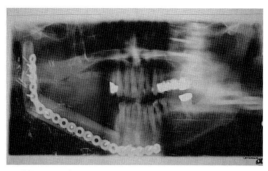

Fig. 7. Radiograph of fibula flap reconstruction of a right mandible with poor height compared with a dentate contralateral mandible.

techniques to increase the fibula's height have been proposed, such as distraction osteogenesis of the segments or "double barreling" of the fibula (**Fig. 8**), but a relatively simple technique is to simply adapt the fibula to abut the native mandible in a slightly more superior position than the inferior border (**Fig. 9**). Of course, a slight cosmetic deformity with a lack of bone at the inferior border may occur, but this deformity is generally minor and of little concern to most patients.

Presurgical planning with the restoring prosthodontist is mandatory before implant surgery. A surgical guide can be fabricated based on the prosthodontist's estimation of the location of the reconstructed bone and his/her ideal locations for implant fixtures. In some cases, this guide may not be helpful because of inaccurate estimation of the bone location but can serve as a blueprint for the next-best implant location. Cone beam computed tomographic scans and implant planning software help mitigate these limitations in the planning phase.

The actual implant placement procedure is no different from that in traditional implant surgery; however, a few principles should be followed. When accessing the implantation sites, if a skin paddle exists over the flap or graft, care should be exercised to preserve the perforator to the skin when designing the incision. Skin paddle revascularization from the surrounding mucosa is unpredictable at best, and at present, there is no way to determine if the skin paddle will survive without its native blood supply. In most mandibular reconstructions, these perforators emerge from the ligual aspect of the reconstructed mandible as is the case with the fibula osteoseptocutaneous flap, iliac crest osteocutaneous flap, and pectoralis major myocutaneous

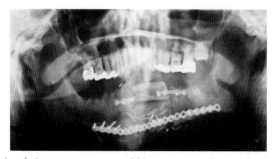

Fig. 8. Radiograph of short-segment mandible reconstruction with double-barrel fibula flap.

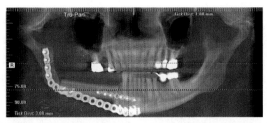

Fig. 9. Radiograph of right mandible reconstruction, with fibula placed slightly superior to the inferior border and secured with a miniplate to more closely approximate the alveolar bone height of the dentate mandible.

flaps placed before free bone grafting of the mandible. Therefore, the incision should be made at the skin-mucosa interface on the lateral or buccal aspect of the skin paddle. This incision allows lingual retraction of the skin paddle and provides access to the bone and fixation hardware. Some circumstances may require the perforators to emerge laterally to the mandible, so careful review of the operative report should be done before implant surgery.

Similar to mandibular reconstruction, if a fibula osteoseptocutaneous flap is used for maxillary reconstruction, often, the perforator to the skin emerges from the palatal aspect of the skin paddle. Again, the incision is made on the lateral aspect of the skin to preserve this blood supply and minimize the risk of devitalizing the skin (**Fig. 10**).

Once the bone is exposed, a minimal amount of periosteal stripping should be performed to preserve as much vascular supply to the neomandible as possible. Implant placement should be avoided in the osteotomy sites because healing may be somewhat incomplete and successful integration of the implants may be compromised (**Fig. 11**). The minimum dimension of an implant is generally considered to be 3.5 mm in diameter and 10 mm in length. With this in mind, the minimum dimension of the reconstruction must be 5.5 mm in width and 10 mm in height. In a study by Frodel and colleagues,[8] the dimensions of cadaveric specimens of several bone flap harvest sites were compared. The bone from the iliac crest and fibula were found to have consistently adequate bone dimensions for implantation based on the similar

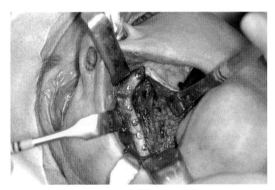

Fig. 10. Implants placed into fibula reconstruction of right maxillectomy defect. The incision to access the fibula is made through the buccal aspect of the skin paddle because of the palatal location of the perforators.

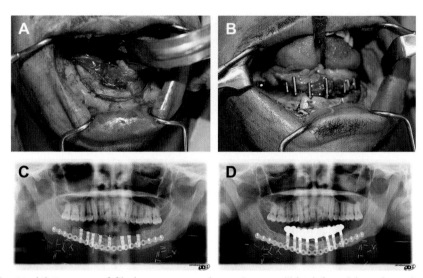

Fig. 11. (*A*) Exposure of fibula-reconstructed anterior mandible defect. (*B*) Implant placement into fibula and native mandible, avoiding the osteotomy and fibula-mandible interface sites. (*C*) Radiograph taken immediately after implant placement. (*D*) Radiograph of fixed prostheses.

minimum dimensions as noted earlier. Although implantation may be possible with other bone harvest sites (scapula, radius), the adequacy of their dimensions is variable.

TIMING OF IMPLANTS

Implants are most commonly placed secondarily into reconstructed jaws, but several investigators advocate implant placement at the time of the initial surgery for reconstruction in cases of benign tumor resections.[9] However, many patients who undergo reconstructive surgery for malignant disease require postoperative radiation therapy. Although the free tissue reconstructed jaw can withstand radiation therapy quite well, there is no consensus regarding the placement of dental implants before or after radiation therapy. On one hand, if implants are placed secondarily, radiation treatment theoretically predisposes these patients to complications, including implant failure, wound dehiscence, and osteoradionecrosis. Although several reports have shown favorable implant success rates in reconstructed jaws exposed to radiation,[10,11] these studies predictably show a lower survival rate for implants in irradiated than in nonirradiated reconstructed jaws. In a review by Teoh and colleagues,[12] the survival rate for implants placed in nonirradiated fibula flaps was 99%, whereas the rate for those placed in irradiated flaps was 92%. Some studies have suggested the use of HBO therapy to improve the success of osteointegration in these patients[13]; however, there have been several reports refuting the efficacy of HBO treatment.[11,14] Specifically, Schoen and colleagues[15] suggested that there was no statistical difference in implant survival in their randomized groups of patients treated with HBO and those not treated with HBO receiving anterior mandibular implants. Of 26 patients, osteoradionecrosis occurred in 1 patient who received HBO therapy.

Placement of implants at the time of the primary reconstructive surgery also has its potential problems, including the possibility of recurrence of the cancer, interference with radiation treatment, potential for poor implant position, and increased duration of surgery. In a simulation study, Friedrich and colleagues[16] simulated an external radiation source aimed at a titanium implant and measured the dose of radiation in the immediate surrounding tissue. Results revealed a 16% reduction of radiation dose directly behind the implant and an 8% increase in dose in the areas immediately in front of and next to the implant. It was concluded that considerable scatter of external radiation occurs with titanium implants and the increased dose at the implant-bone interface may affect bone healing or lead to osteoradionecrosis. Furthermore, De Ceulaer and colleagues,[17] in a recent review of 21 patients who received implants either primarily during the initial surgery or secondarily, found 3 cancer recurrences in the mucosa directly surrounding the implants. All 3 recurrences occurred in patients who had implants placed primarily. The investigators stated that no conclusions can be made because of the small sample size, but this study indicates that the risk of recurrence is real, although not quantifiable at present.

In secondary implant placement, no consensus exists for how long an interval is ideal between the primary reconstructive surgery and implant placement. However, some studies recommend a period of 1 year after cancer surgery to allow for complete bone healing, improved nutritional status, and monitoring of disease recurrence.[9,18] In benign disease, implant reconstruction can proceed once it is determined that bone healing has been achieved (usually between 4 and 6 months).

Finally, there is debate as to whether dental reconstruction is even necessary in the patient with cancer. In a review of 28 patients who underwent prosthetic reconstruction, Leung and Cheung[19] revealed that only 32% of the patients had no limitations of food consistency and 28.6% had problems associated with prosthetic instability. Indeed, many patients with a successful bone and soft tissue reconstruction of their jaws do not desire further dental reconstruction. In the available literature, rates of full dental rehabilitation in patients with cancer can vary (20%–100%).[8,9,20–22] This variation can be explained by the nature of the retrospective case series patient selection bias that makes up the bulk of the literature. In the authors' own informal case series, only 20% with tumor who underwent bone reconstruction have gone on to have dental implants. In the United States, with poor medical insurance coverage for dental implants, the most obvious obstacle is the cost of treatment. However, in research from countries where these services are covered through national health plans, there are still a significant number of patients who do not opt for dental rehabilitation. Obviously, several factors can influence a patient's decision of not to seek dental rehabilitation. Many patients are able function adequately without dental prosthetics, with only minor limitations of food intake.

MANAGEMENT OF SOFT TISSUE

Ablative surgery for oral cancer generally requires excision of the attached gingival tissue. This tissue, which is tightly adherent to the underlying bone, has the ideal characteristics for implant emergence. The nature of the attached gingiva provides immobile tissue around implant abutments and ease of oral hygiene to prevent periimplantitis (**Fig. 12**). Unfortunately, the soft tissues imported with various reconstruction techniques do not adequately replicate the unique properties of keratinized gingiva. The skin paddles of osteocutaneous flaps provide the necessary tissue to close oral wounds and allow separation of the mouth and neck during the initial healing of the flap. However, the thick, mobile nature of this tissue is a poor medium for implant emergence.

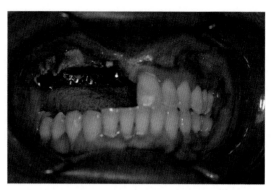

Fig. 12. Periimplantitis around the framework of implant-stabilized maxillary prosthesis of the fibula-reconstructed maxilla.

Several techniques are available to address these issues. First, thinning of the skin paddle can be performed at any phase of the implant treatment plan. The authors prefer to perform this procedure at the time of second-stage surgery rather than at implant placement to assure adequate soft tissue coverage of the bone and implants at the time of placement. Thinning can be done in a traditional open method or with aggressive liposuction as described by Holmes and Aponte-Wesson.[23] In lieu of flap thinning, or if no skin paddle is present, a vestibuloplasty can be performed with split-thickness skin (**Fig. 13**). Vestibuloplasty can also be performed with second-stage surgery or as a separate procedure. A custom-fabricated splint should be used for several weeks to allow firm adaptation to the reconstructed jaw. This procedure can also address the common lack of vestibule depth that occurs after many reconstructions.

Unfortunately, these measures often fail to prevent periimplantitis for several reasons. First, the area is often insensate and the patient does not have the proprioception necessary to perform adequate oral hygiene. Second, the nature of the dental reconstruction can make hygiene difficult for many patients because of the presence of implant abutments and prosthetic suprastructures. Generally, hyperplastic tissues surrounding implants should be excised periodically and professional oral hygiene performed on a frequent and regular basis. Localized areas can be addressed with

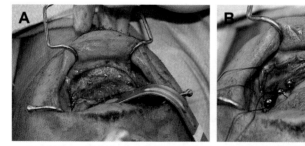

Fig. 13. (A) Second-stage surgery of implant placed into fibula-reconstructed mandible. Supraperiosteal dissection performed for vestibuloplasty. (B) Split-thickness skin placed over the fibula to gain vestibule depth and fixed tissue surrounding implants. This setup is secured with a custom-fabricated acrylic splint for a period of 3 to 4 weeks.

palatal grafts, or larger areas can be skin grafted again in an attempt to obtain fixed, keratinized tissue around implant interfaces.

SUMMARY

Use of dental implants in oral cancer reconstruction has become an important aspect of the reconstructive plan for these patients. With improvements in technology and sophistication in prosthesis fabrication, extremely functional and cosmetic outcomes can be achieved. The future of dental rehabilitation in patients with cancer holds much promise and can positively affect patients' quality of life with improved function and cosmesis. It is still a long, multistage process for patients to endure, but the end result can potentially allow patients to minimize the consequences, limitations, and stigmata of ablative cancer surgery.

REFERENCES

1. Niimi A, Ueda M, Kaneda T. Maxillary obturator supported by osseointegrated implants placed in irradiated bone: report of cases. J Oral Maxillofac Surg 1993;51:804–9.
2. Salinas T, Sadan A, Peterson T, et al. Zygomaticus implants: a new treatment for the edentulous maxilla. Quintessence Dent Technol 2001;24:171–80.
3. Schmidt BL, Pogrel MA, Young CW, et al. Reconstruction of extensive maxillary defects using zygomaticus implants. J Oral Maxillofac Surg 2004;62(Suppl 2): 82–9.
4. Hirsch DL, Howell KL, Levine JP. A novel approach to palatomaxillary reconstruction: use of radial forearm free tissue transfer combined with zygomaticus implants. J Oral Maxillofac Surg 2009;67:2466–72.
5. Zwahlen RA, Grätz KW, Oechslin CK, et al. Survival rate of zygomatic implants in atrophic or partially resected maxillae prior to functional loading: a retrospective clinical report. Int J Oral Maxillofac Implants 2006;21:413–20.
6. Marx RE, Ames JR. The use of hyperbaric oxygen therapy in bony reconstruction of the irradiated and tissue-deficient patient. J Oral Maxillofac Surg 1982;40: 412–20.
7. Hidalgo DA. Fibula free flap: a new method of mandible reconstruction. Plast Reconstr Surg 1989;84:71–9.
8. Frodel JL, Funk GF, Capper DT, et al. Osseointegrated implants: a comparative study of bone thickness in four vascularized bone flaps. Plast Reconstr Surg 1993;92:449–55.
9. Chana JS, Chang YM, Wei FC, et al. Segmental mandibulectomy and immediate free fibula osteoseptocutaneous flap reconstruction with endosseous implants: an ideal treatment method for mandibular ameloblastoma. Plast Reconstr Surg 2004;113:80–7.
10. Adell R, Svensson B, Bågenholm T. Dental rehabilitation in 101 primarily reconstructed jaws after segmental resections – possibilities and problems. An 18-year study. J Craniomaxillofac Surg 2008;36:395–402.
11. Cuesta-Gil M, Caicoya SO, Riba-Garcia F, et al. Oral rehabilitation with osseointegrated implants in oncologic patients. J Oral Maxillofac Surg 2009;67:2485–96.
12. Teoh KH, Huryn JM, Patel S, et al. Implant prosthodontic rehabilitation of fibula free-flap reconstructed mandible: a Memorial Sloan-Kettering Cancer Center review of prognostic factors and implant outcomes. Int J Oral Maxillofac Implants 2005;20:738–46.

13. Barber HD, Seckinger RJ, Hayden RE, et al. Evaluation of osseointegration of endosseous implants in radiated, vascularized fibula flaps to the mandible: a pilot study. J Oral Maxillofac Surg 1995;53:640–4.

14. Eckert SE, Desjardins RP, Keller EE, et al. Endosseous implants in an irradiated tissue bed. J Prosthet Dent 1996;76:45–9.

15. Schoen PJ, Raghoeber GM, Bouma J, et al. Rehabilitation of oral function in head and neck cancer patients after radiotherapy with implant retained dentures: effects of hyperbaric oxygen therapy. Oral Oncol 2007;43:379–88.

16. Friedrich RE, Todrovic M, Krüll A. Simulation of scattering effects of irradiation on surroundings using the example of titanium dental implants: a Monte Carlo approach. Anticancer Res 2010;30:1727–30.

17. De Ceulaer J, Magremanne M, van Veen A, et al. Squamous cell carcinoma recurrence around dental implants. J Oral Maxillofac Surg 2010;68:2507–12.

18. Jacobson M, Tjellstrom A, Albrektsson T, et al. Integration of titanium implants in irradiated bone. Histologic and clinical study. Ann Otol Rhinol Laryngol 1988;97:337–40.

19. Leung AC, Cheung LK. Dental implants in reconstructed jaws: patients' evaluation of functional and quality-of-life outcomes. Int J Oral Maxillofac Implants 2003;18:127–34.

20. Rogers SN, Panasar J, Pritchard K, et al. Survey of oral rehabilitation in a consecutive series of 130 patients treated by primary resection for oral and oropharyngeal squamous cell carcinoma. Br J Oral Maxillofac Surg 2005;43:23–30.

21. Anthony JP, Foster RD, Kaplan JM, et al. Fibular free flap reconstruction of the "true" lateral mandibular defect. Ann Plast Surg 1997;38:137–46.

22. Weischer T, Mohr C. Ten-year experience in oral rehabilitation of cancer patients: treatment concepts and proposed criteria for success. Int J Oral Maxillofac Implants 1999;14:521–8.

23. Holmes JD, Aponte-Wesson R. Dental implants after reconstruction with free tissue transfer. Oral Maxillofac Surg Clin North Am 2010;22:407–18.

Dental Implants and the Use of rhBMP-2

Daniel B. Spagnoli, MS, PhD, DDS[a],*, Robert E. Marx, DDS[b]

KEYWORDS

• Dental implant • Tissue engineering • rhBMP-2
• Bone morphogenetic proteins • de-novo bone regeneration

Congenital deformity, oral diseases, trauma, and tumors are all causes of missing teeth.[1,2] Tooth loss interferes with the ability to chew and speak and reduces confidence in social interactions. Missing teeth ultimately diminish an individual's nutritional, physical, social, and psychological quality of life.[3–7]

Tissue engineering is an emerging field of medicine and dentistry that combines the body's natural biologic response to tissue injury with engineering principles. Tissue engineering principles are based on a philosophy of recruiting or combining mesenchymal stem cells with form and attachment to provide constructs that carry chemotactic, proliferative, and inductive growth factors. The goal of this strategy is to replicate or reconstruct the natural form and function of missing tissues and organs. Rapid progress in the field of tissue-engineered tooth regeneration suggests that this will eventually become a reality.[8] Tissue-engineered bone with native qualities will be necessary for implantation or migration of engineered teeth in the future, and is currently required for the osseointegration of dental implants.

Experts now recognize that functional and esthetic results obtained with dental implants are optimized when reverse engineering principals are used during the treatment planning phase of patient care. Radiographs, including CT scans; treatment planning software; stereolithographic models; and dental models are used to supplement the clinical examination of the patient. Together the prosthodontist, or restorative dentist, and the oral and maxillofacial surgeon formulate a prosthetic-driven restorative plan for patients. The surgeon must then determine the best approach to engineering bone that is vital, with normal vascular, cortical, trabecular, and marrow components, to replace the native anatomy needed for the planned implants. Bone graft techniques must be chosen based on knowledge of mechanisms of bone

This article was previously published in the May 2011 issue of *Oral and Maxillofacial Surgery Clinics of North America*.

[a] University Oral and Maxillofacial Surgery, 8738 University City Boulevard, Charlotte, NC 28213, USA
[b] Division of Oral and Maxillofacial Surgery, University of Miami School of Medicine, Deering Medical Plaza, 9380 SW 150th Street, Suite 190, Miami, FL 33157, USA
* Corresponding author.
E-mail address: dspagnoli@uomsnc.com

Dent Clin N Am 55 (2011) 883–907
doi:10.1016/j.cden.2011.07.014
0011-8532/11/$ – see front matter © 2011 Elsevier Inc. All rights reserved.

regeneration and attachment to implant surfaces. A review of bone grafts and graft substitutes applied to guided bone regeneration suggested that autogenous bone or bone graft substitutes used in areas where implants are placed should be completely resorbed and replaced by the formation of new bone so that implants can be placed in vital bone alone.[9]

This article addresses the role of bone morphogenetic proteins (BMP) in native bone healing for implant attachments and the application of BMP to de novo bone regeneration associated with dental implants.

BACKGROUND

During the 1950s, the initial observations of titanium osseointegration into bone were made by Brånemark.[10] These observations were not made during research to discover a bone implant, but instead during in vivo vital microscopy studies of bone marrow microvasculature. To perform these studies, Brånemark developed in vivo bone microscopy chambers based on the principals of those used in rabbit ears or hamster cheek pouches to study microvasculature. The chambers were threaded titanium cylinders with a hollow central canal and a lateral transverse opening that could be threaded into bone. When these chambers were placed in bone, vessels from the marrow space would grow into the central chamber, allowing the circulation within bone marrow and the role of blood vessels during bone healing to be studied with in vivo microscopy.

During this research, Brånemark discovered that the titanium chambers became fused to the bone and could not be removed without fracturing the bone. Brånemark introduced the term *osseointegration* to describe the concept of stable fixation of titanium to bone, and determined that this concept could be useful in designing dental and orthopedic prosthetic anchors.[11,12] An important consideration derived from these early observations is that the vascular and vital nature of the bone is essential for the cascade of events that leads to osseointegration.

Osseointegration has been extensively studied and can be considered an anchorage between biomaterial and vital bone.[13–15] Currently, an implant is considered osseointegrated when no progressive relative movement occurs between the implant and bone. Many factors affect the strength and rate of osseointegration, including implant surface geometry, surface chemistry, nature of and technique for host site preparation, and degree of stress or strain on the implant during the early phases of osseointegration.[16,17] Although osseointegration is usually considered an attachment between bone and metals, such as titanium or zirconium, it is actually an attachment between bone and a metal oxide layer, with a thin interposed proteoglycan layer. Titanium reacts with oxygen to form a titanium dioxide (TIO_2) layer that changes the surface properties to become highly polarized. The polarized surface attracts water-soluble molecules and binds polyvalent cations, which form a negative charge on the implant surface. Soluble calcium ions become attached to the TIO_2 surface through electrostatic interactions and bind proteins and proteoglycans to the implant oxide surface.

The quality of osseous regeneration within the implant–bone interface zone and tissue attachment to the implant depends on bone vascularity and osteogenic potential. Bone, and especially the marrow space adjacent to an implant site, is the source of stem cells, growth and differentiation factors, soluble bone and plasma proteins, and vessels that contribute to the bone healing response.[18] Endosseous implants become integrated to bone through three mechanisms, including osteoconduction, de novo bone formation, and bone remodeling.

Bone regeneration and attachment to an implant surface follows a mixture of two different pathways, termed *distance* and *contact osteogenesis*.[19] In distance osteogenesis, bone regeneration extends through appositional deposition from the surface of the bone osteotomy toward the surface of the implant. A blood clot, including fibrin and platelets, forms within the gap and a process typical of bone healing follows.[20,21] An inflammatory response, including monocytes, leads to the development of osteoclasts that attach to damaged bone surfaces. BMP-2 receptors are located on monocytes, and BMP-2 has been shown to be chemotactic for monocytes.

Osteocalcin within the extracellular matrix of exposed bone acts as a signal that influences osteoclast differentiation.[22] Osteoclasts migrate and attach to bone surfaces through an integrin-mediated process, in which they form a sealing zone called a *Howship's lacunae*. Osteoclasts secrete acids and hydrolytic enzymes, leading to localized surface resorption of bone and exposure of the extracellular matrix of bone that contains BMPs. Osteoprogenitor cells are recruited from marrow, periosteum, or pericytes associated with repair vessels and differentiate on existing bone surfaces. Osteoblasts then form new matrix and osteoid, leading to trabecular bone apposition that fills the osteotomy gap and attaches to the implant surface. This form of osseointegration attachment is characterized by a layer of cells interposed between the bone matrix and the implant surface.

Contact osteogenesis relies more on processes consistent with de novo bone formation. Surgical drilling and bone preparation for implant placement results in a cascade of events that mimic normal bone healing. The implant surface is initially coated with blood and plasma proteins that become adsorbed to the implant surface. Fibrin in the healing site becomes adherent to implant surfaces and acts as an early matrix for cells participating in the inflammatory process of wound healing. Platelets almost immediately attach to the implant surface, followed by platelet activation and the release of cytokines and growth factors within the osteotomy implant gap.[23]

Fibrin retention and platelet activation are enhanced by implant surfaces with greater microtexture. Neutrophils become attached to the titanium surface and are subsequently activated. Activated neutrophils produce reactive oxygen at the implant surface through membrane-bound NADPH oxidase and thus may play a role in secondary oxidation of the implant surface. Neutrophils function as phagocytes, and at maturation undergo autolysis and release inflammatory cytokines, including prostaglandins and leukotrienes. Monocytes located within blood clots attach to implant surfaces via an integrin-mediated association with serum fibronectin and vitonectin.[24] Monocytes differentiate into macrophages that attach to titanium oxide surfaces through $\beta 1$ integrins, a function that is improved by an enhanced microtexture. Macrophages further contribute to the implant surface niche by secreting bone sialoprotein and osteopontin factors associated with bone mineralization.[25] Implant surface attached macrophages also contribute to implant-related de novo bone formation through stimulating osteoinduction via the synthesis and secretion of platelet-derived growth factor β (PDFG-β) and BMP-2.[26]

Therefore, titanium implant osseointegration involves in situ physical chemical and biologic modification of the implant surface. In distance osseointegration, osteoclastic resorption of bone surfaces exposes the bone extracellular matrix and BMP, leading to osteogenesis and appositional bone development in the direction of the implant. In contact osseointegration, macrophages attach to conditioned implant surfaces and synthesize and secrete BMPs. Both processes probably exist in most cases of implant placement, and thus the monocyte-derived macrophages and osteoclasts play a pivotal role in BMP-mediated de novo bone formation for implant attachment.

Basic principles of BMP mechanisms of action are similar for host-derived or implanted BMPs and are discussed as a common subject. BMPs are members of the transforming growth factor-β superfamily of growth factors.[27] They are key regulators of cellular growth and differentiation, and regulate tissue formation in both developing and mature organisms. Twenty unique BMP ligands have been identified and categorized into subclasses based on amino acid sequence similarity.[28–33] BMPs are synthesized inside of cells as precursor proteins with N-linked glycosylation sites, a hydrophobic secretory leader, and a propeptide sequence joined to the mature region, which forms dimers with other BMPs. The mature segment of BMPs is located at the carboxy terminal and contains seven cysteine amino acid residues. Six of the amino acids are involved in the formation of intrachain disulphide bonds that form a rigid cysteine-knot molecular structure. The seventh cysteine residue is involved in the formation of dimers via an interchain disulphide bond.

BMPs exposed within or secreted into a wound affect mesenchymal stem cell (MSC) accumulation through chemotaxis and proliferation; however, PDGF-β, which is also secreted by macrophages, has a more potent chemotactic and proliferation effect on MSCs.[34] Sources of MSCs include bone marrow, periosteum, pericytes, and circulating MSCs. MSCs are influenced by BMP-2 to differentiate either directly into osteoblasts for intramembranous bone development or into chondrocytes, followed by cartilage development and removal for endochondral bone formation. Osteoinductive activities of BMPs on MSCs are elicited through transmembrane serine/threonine kinase–type receptors unique to the tumor necrosis factor β superfamily of growth factors. BMP-2 interacts with the type I receptor BMPR1A and the type II receptor BMPR2. Binding of the BMP-2 dimers to the types I and II serine/threonine kinase receptors results in the formation of a heterotetramer-activated receptor complex and activation of the signaling cascade. Immediately after binding, the type II receptor kinase phosphorylates the type I receptor. In turn, the type I receptor phosphorylates the intracytoplasmic signaling molecules receptor-Smads 1 and 5.

Smad proteins are one of the BMPR1 substrates, and play a critical second messenger type of role in relaying BMP signals from receptors to target genes to the nucleus. After receptor-Smads 1 and 5 are phosphorylated, activated receptor-Smads are released from their receptors and combine with Smad 4 a Co-Smad or common mediator Smad. This combination forms hetero-oligomeric complexes. These complexes are then translocated to the nucleus to interact with transcription factors to mediate target gene activation.

Runx-2 is the essential transcription factor for BMP response genes. It belongs to the Runt family of transcription factors and plays a critical role in determining the osteoblast cell lineage and initiating osteoblast differentiation.[35] Runx-2 expression also regulates bone extracellular matrix protein genes that encode for bone sialoprotein, osteocalcin, and type I collagen, and could therefore be a downstream target of cellular events such as extracellular matrix adhesion–mediated signaling, changes in cell shape, and responses to stress. Osterix is a second transcription factor, which may play a key role in perpetuating differentiation along the osteogenic versus chondrogenic pathway, which may be significant in development or regeneration of intramembranous bone.[36]

Vascularization is observed at the transition of preosteoblasts to mature osteoblasts during both development and fracture-healing. BMP-induced vascular endothelial growth factor α (VEGF-α) production in osteoblasts plays an important role in the coupling of bone formation and angiogenesis by acting as a chemoattractant for neighboring endothelial cells and stimulating VEGF-α secretion by osteoblasts and endothelial cells.[37–39] Vascular proliferation in relationship to preosteoblast condensations during de novo bone formation underscores the transition from MSCs that can survive with low oxygen tensions to osteoblasts that require high oxygen tension.

Before differentiation, osteoblast precursor cells must form integrin-mediated attachments with extracellular matrix molecules. Integrins are transmembrane receptors that interact with attachment peptide sequences of extracellular space molecules that contain an arginine-glycine-asparagine terminal.[40] This terminal sequence, referred to as RGD, is found on numerous extracellular matrix proteins, including fibrin, collagen, fibronectin, vitronectin, osteopontin, and bone sialoprotein. Preosteoblast contact guidance on extracellular matrix proteins is integrin-mediated, and osteoblasts establish crosstalk with the extracellular matrix via integrins.[41,42] Intricate attachment plaques develop from microtubules and other peptides within the osteoblast cytoplasm at integrin sites, and transfer information regarding extracellular matrix stress and strain to the nucleus, resulting in synthesis and secretion of osseous development or maintenance matrix.

Osteoblast differentiation results in the formation of cuboidal-shaped cells with organelles capable of synthesis and secretion of all components of bone. These cells are polarized with their nucleus toward the upper part of the cell and their protein synthetic apparatus toward the extracellular matrix. Osteoblasts initiate bone formation through secreting osteoid, an unmineralized bone matrix. Osteoblasts then secrete apatite minerals and alkaline phosphatase located within special secretory vesicles called *matrix vesicles*. The contents of matrix vesicles interact with collagen and other extracellular matrix proteins to form mineralized matrix. Osteoblasts become surrounded by their mineralized matrix and become osteocytes. Early bone formation is less organized and referred to as *woven bone*. Stress and strain forces lead to osteoclast-mediated remodeling and the eventual formation of mature bone, identified by the organization of Haversian systems, which are the functional units of bone. Bone formation eventually results in the formation of cortical trabecular and marrow components.

The only BMP currently available for grafting of maxillofacial implant sites is recombinant human BMP-2 (rhBMP-2). The BMP-2 is marketed by Medtronic Biologics as Infuse, a device available in various kit sizes that include lyophilized rhBMP2, a diluent, and an acellular collagen sponge (ACS) carrier/matrix. The rh-BMP2 is reconstituted with the diluent and then applied to the ACS at a 1.5-mg/mL concentration with a collagen binding time of 15 minutes before use. Significant preclinical testing and human clinical controlled trials led to its approval,[43–45] and are reviewed elsewhere.[46]

Histologic specimens were obtained with a trephine technique used at implant placement during the clinical trials. The findings of the histologic assessment showed development of native bone through a de novo intramembranous pathway that replicates native bone development. Preosteoblast condensations were observed in association with blood vessels, and osteoblasts were observed forming new bone trabeculae through appositional secretion of osteoid and mineralized matrix. Osteoclast remodeling of the trabeculae was also observed. Mature bone had normal Haversian systems within trabeculae and regenerated normal vascular cellular marrow spaces. **Figs. 1–4** are from rhBMP-2 graft specimens obtained from the sinus lift human clinical trial, and show stages of de novo intramembranous bone formation.[8,47]

The use of BMP-2 is now well founded for the sinus floor grafting indication, as seen in a recent clinical case (**Figs. 5–14**) in which combined alveolar and sinus augmentation was performed in conjunction with simultaneous implant placement. Performance of all three of these procedures at one time is facilitated by the bone regenerative power of this biologic agent.

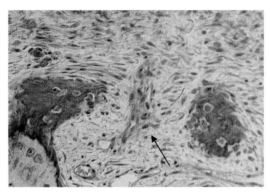

Fig. 1. Early-stage de novo bone formation: the arrow points to a condensation of preosteo-blasts in a vascular field.

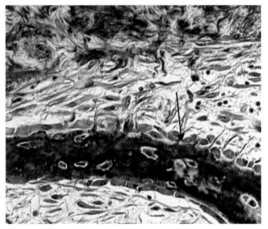

Fig. 2. Early formation of trabecular bone. Arrow points to osteoblast appositional deposition of osteoid.

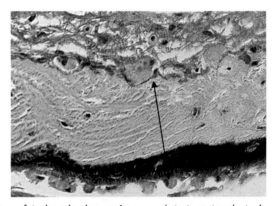

Fig. 3. Remodeling of trabecular bone. Arrow points to osteoclast above and osteoblast below.

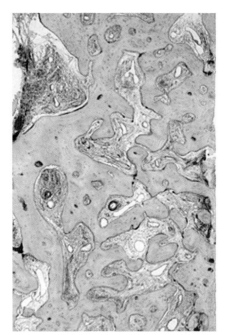

Fig. 4. A trephine specimen of mature regenerated bone with viable and vascular trabeculae and marrow with no residual debris. (*Modified from* Triplett RG, Nevins M, Marx RE, et al. Pivotal randomized, parallel evaluation of recombinant human bone morphogenetic protein-2/absorbable collagen sponge and autogenous bone graft for maxillary sinus floor augmentation. J Oral Maxillofac Surg 2009;67:1947–60; with permission.)

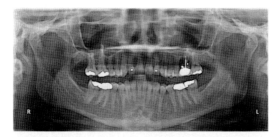

Fig. 5. Failed root canal therapy in upper left first molar with abscess.

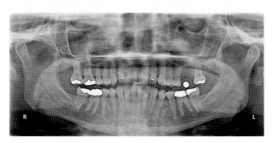

Fig. 6. Postextraction shows a vertical ridge deficiency and slight ridge width deficit.

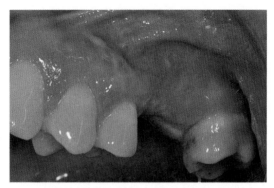

Fig. 7. Residual ridge 2 months postextraction. Note tissue discoloration from previous apicoectomy and retrofill.

Bone preparation and implant placement results in modification of the implant surface to permit interactions with osteoblasts and bone extracellular matrix molecules that mimic normal bone healing. BMPs are involved at multiple steps of this progression both naturally and now as a graft component. The availability of Infuse provides surgeons with a method of grafting that allows the engineering of bone before implant placement that meets the requirements alluded to earlier for native cellular vascular bone with no residual inert components. Bone that is viable with normal marrow and trabeculae not only provides a natural matrix for implant stability but also permits the establishment of an extracellular matrix–to–integrin–to–cell relationship essential for bone maintenance.

TRANSLATIONAL RESEARCH: THE CLINICAL APPLICATION OF COMPLEX BIOLOGIC STUDIES

Clinical use of the complex mechanism of bone regeneration from rhBMP-2 distills down to completing the classic tissue engineering triangle consisting of a source of cells, a signal, and a matrix (scaffold) on which bone can form (**Fig. 15**). In other words,

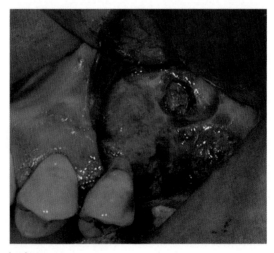

Fig. 8. Sinus lift osteotomy.

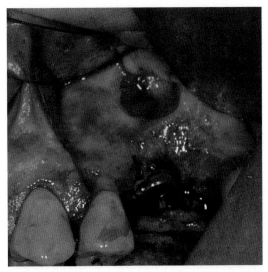

Fig. 9. XX small Infuse rhBMP-2/ACS graft placed in sinus floor and simultaneous implant placement; 2 mm of the facial surface of the implant remains exposed.

liquid rhBMP squirted into a site will not regenerate much and likely no bone at all, and even rhBMP-2/ACS alone has shown little bone regeneration in larger defects because the ACS is 90% air, which is an inadequate scaffold in larger-volume defects (**Fig. 16**).

The following two cases will illustrate the translation of a complex biology involving rhBMP-2/ACS, crushed cancellous freeze-dried allogeneic bone (CCFDAB), and

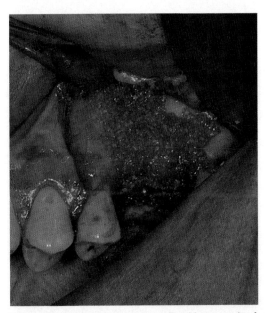

Fig. 10. Particulate allogeneic freeze-dried demineralized bone and Infuse mix packed over the lateral surface.

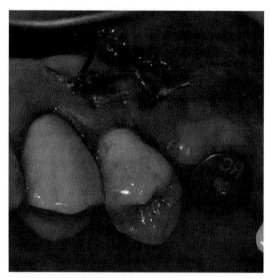

Fig. 11. One week after graft and implant placement.

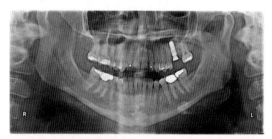

Fig. 12. Five months after graft and implant with excellent consolidation of graft.

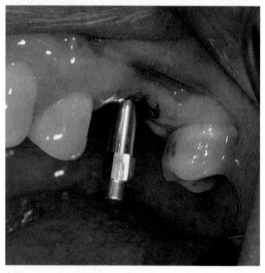

Fig. 13. Implant stability quotient at 5 months after graft and implant was 75 × 77.

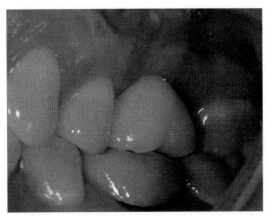

Fig. 14. The implant is functionally restored. Total treatment time from graft and implant placement to final restoration was 6 months.

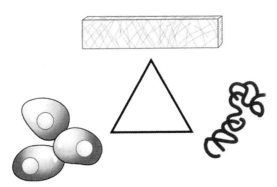

Fig. 15. The classic tissue engineering triangle required to regenerate lost tissues.

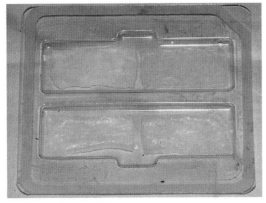

Fig. 16. The acellular collagen sponge is not highly cross-linked and therefore has 90% air spaces.

platelet-rich plasma (PRP) into a predictable bone regeneration that provides a functional benefit to patients through the osseointegration of dental implants. In these cases, the rhBMP-2/ACS and the growth factors in PRP provide the signal, and the host bone surface, the PRP, and the rhBMP-2 each provide a source of cells through a different mechanism. That is, the host bone provides contact osteogenesis through the migration of osteoblasts and local osteoprogenitor stem cells; the PRP provides a concentrated number of stem cells from the peripheral blood; and the rhBMP-2 provides stem cells from the blood through its inherent chemoattraction. Finally, the CCFDAB provides a rough surface for bone formation, and the PRP cell adhesion molecules together provide the matrix on which bone can regenerate, thus completing the tissue engineering triangle. This type of bone regeneration represents in situ tissue engineering.

Case 1: Complete Vertical Augmentation of the Maxilla

A 61-year-old man with a severe loss of maxillary alveolar bone height and width resulting from early maxillary tooth loss, but with retention of his native mandibular teeth, presented with a complete arch combination syndrome (**Figs. 17** and **18**). The reconstruction began with a midcrestal incision and mucoperiosteal flap reflections of the buccal and palatal mucosa, exposing a small and severely thin (knife-edge) ridge (**Fig. 19**). A titanium mesh was fabricated to contain and protect the graft and to shape an ideal ridge (**Fig. 20**), and 12 mg of rhBMP-2/ACS at 1.5 mg/mL concentration was placed on the ACS and allowed to bond for more than 15 minutes (**Fig. 21**). Furthermore, 7 mL of PRP was developed by harvesting 60 mL of autologous blood and processing it into a concentrate using a double-spin centrifuge with a floating shelf canister specific to the density of platelets (**Fig. 22**). CCFDAB was obtained as a sterilized graft particulate from the University of Miami Tissue Bank (**Fig. 23**). The PRP was activated with four drops of a mixture obtained by placing 5 mL of 10% calcium chloride into 5000 units of topical bovine thrombin and mixed into the CCFDAB. The rhBMP-2/ACS was cut into squares, added to the above two materials, and mixed thoroughly to form a composite graft (**Fig. 24**).

The composite graft consisting of 12 mg of rhBMP-2/ACS at a 1:1 ratio with CCFDAB and PRP was placed into the preformed titanium mesh (**Fig. 25**). The mesh was placed into the prepared recipient area and fixed with monocortical screws (**Fig. 26**). The buccal mucosa was extensively undermined to achieve a primary closure (**Fig. 27**).

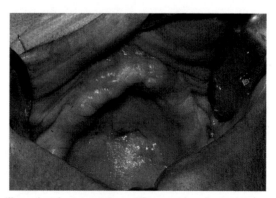

Fig. 17. Total maxillary alveolar resorption with scarred and retracted mucosa from combination syndrome.

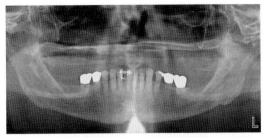

Fig. 18. Radiograph indicating severe maxillary alveolar bone loss from combination syndrome.

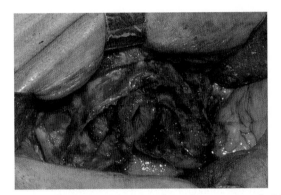

Fig. 19. Knife-edge maxillary alveolar ridge together with severe vertical bone resorption.

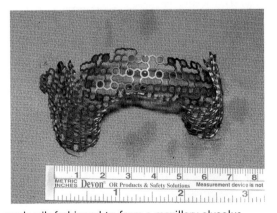

Fig. 20. Titanium mesh crib fashioned to form a maxillary alveolus.

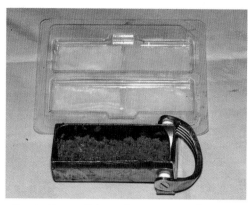

Fig. 21. rhBMP-2 bonding to the acellular collagen sponge for 15 minutes or more before adding to the CCFDAB-PRP composite.

After 6 months of bone maturity, the graft showed significant consolidation on a cone beam CT scan (**Fig. 28**). On reentry, an ideal ridge with more than 1 cm of vertical and 1 cm of horizontal gain was observed (**Fig. 29**) that accommodated nine dental implants (**Fig. 30**). The implants were uncovered 6 months later during a vestibular extension procedure, which eventuated into a milled bar retained denture (**Fig. 31**), which has been functional for the past 2 years.

Case 2: Continuity Defect of the Mandible Salvaging a Deficient-Free Vascular Fibula Graft

A 46-year-old woman who received a free vascular fibula graft for an osteosarcoma was referred by her maxillofacial prosthodontist because a "denture appliance was impossible." Radiographs showed a small straight piece of bone not in the normal plane or curvature of the mandible and with an extremely deficient vertical height (**Fig. 32**). In addition, the proximal segment bearing the condyle and part of the ramus was rotated anteriorly and superiorly. A facial concavity caused by the lingual position of the graft and a severe scarring and deformity of the leg where the fibula was taken were also present (**Fig. 33**).

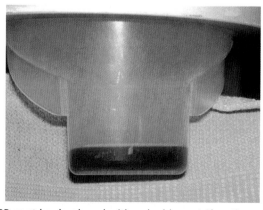

Fig. 22. Quality PRP must be developed with a double centrifugation concept to yield the maximum number of platelets and cell adhesion molecules.

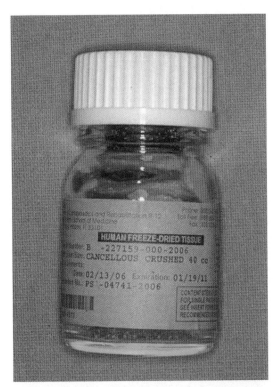

Fig. 23. Crushed cancellous allogeneic bone from the University of Miami Tissue Bank has the appropriate surface characteristics and is guaranteed to be sterile.

Although the initial intent was to reposition the fibula and add graft material to gain vertical height, upon osteomyzing etc the fibula (**Fig. 34**) and repositioning the proximal segment, the fibula was observed to be significantly out of place (**Fig. 35**). The only option was to resect the nonfunctional and deficient fibula and proceed to graft a 9-cm continuity defect (**Fig. 36**). Similar to Case 1, 12 mg of rhBMP-2/ACS was used, as was CCFDAB. However, 10 mL of a bone marrow aspirate concentrate (BMAC) was used rather than PRP; 60 mL of bone marrow was aspirated from the anterior ilium (**Fig. 37**) and concentrated in a double-spin centrifuge with a canister

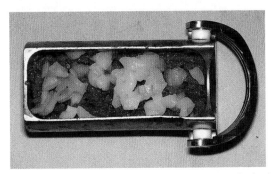

Fig. 24. The rhBMP-2/ACS is best cut into small 1 × 1 cm squares, which are then distributed evenly through the graft material.

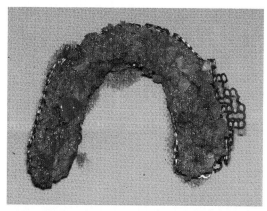

Fig. 25. The graft of 12 mg of rhBMP-2/ACS, at a 1:1 ratio with CCFDAB and PRP, placed into the titanium mesh.

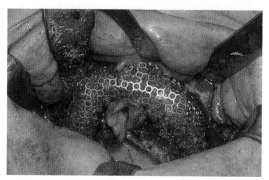

Fig. 26. The titanium mesh containing the composite rhBMP-2/ACS-CCFDAB-PRP graft is placed and fixated with monocortical screws.

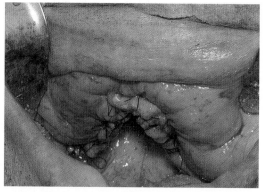

Fig. 27. Significant undermining and advancement of the buccal mucosa is required to gain a tension-free closure.

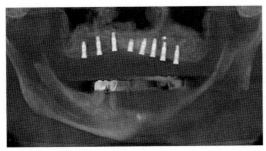

Fig. 28. Excellent bone regeneration and graft consolidation is noted on a 6-month cone-beam CT scan.

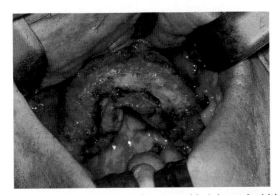

Fig. 29. On reentry, a robust alveolar ridge of improved height and width is noted to have formed.

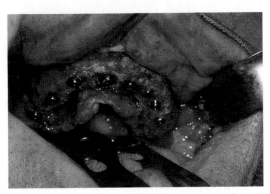

Fig. 30. The newly regenerated ridge was sufficient to accommodate nine dental implants.

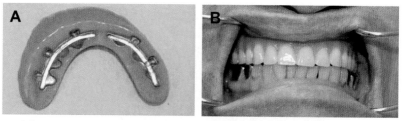

Fig. 31. (*A*) A milled bar maxillary denture was used to rehabilitate the lost dentition. (*B*) Milled bar denture in place and stable after 2 years.

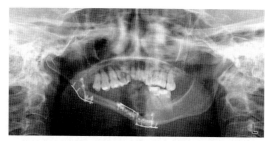

Fig. 32. Fibula reconstruction of mandibular defect with deficient height, morphology, and volume.

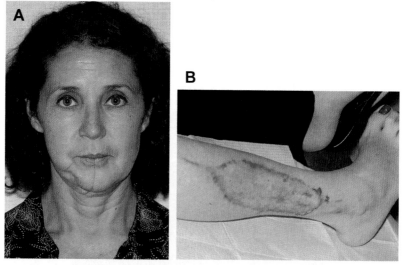

Fig. 33. (*A*) Facial cosmetic deformity caused by straight and small fibula. (*B*) Cosmetic and functional deformity of fibula donor site. This person could not move her great toe and had a general weakness of her foot.

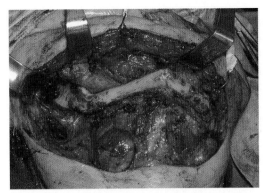

Fig. 34. Fibula healed but is too small and too straight to reconstruct a mandible. Its deficient length also caused a malocclusion and a rotation of the right ramus-condyle segment (see **Fig. 1**).

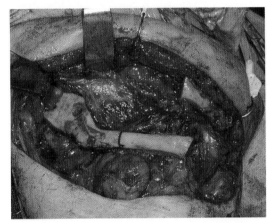

Fig. 35. On sectioning the host bone fibula junction, the proximal segment repositioned, orienting the fibula into an unusable position.

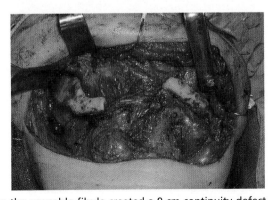

Fig. 36. Removing the unusable fibula created a 9-cm continuity defect.

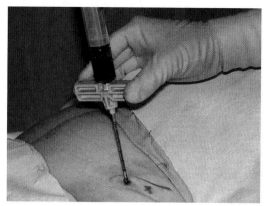

Fig. 37. Osteoprogenitor/stem cells harvested from the anterior ilium via simple aspiration.

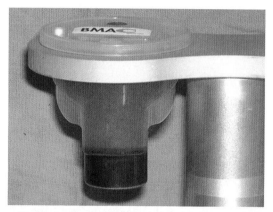

Fig. 38. Osteoprogenitor/stem cells concentrated with the same device used to prepare PRP. This bone marrow aspirate concentrate yielded 7.68×10^6 of CD44+ osteoprogenitor cells.

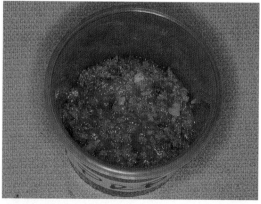

Fig. 39. Composite graft consisting of 12 mg of rhBMP-2/ACS cut into 1×1 cm squares and added to CCFDAB-BMAC.

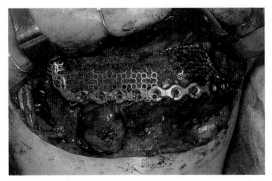

Fig. 40. The composite graft placed into the continuity defect and stabilized with a titanium plate and mesh.

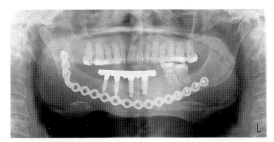

Fig. 41. Excellent bone regeneration created by the rhBMP-2/ACS-CCFDAB-BMAC graft permitted placement of five implants and a denture reconstruction.

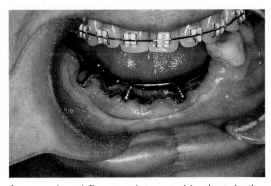

Fig. 42. Hader bar framework and five osseointegrated implants in the mature graft.

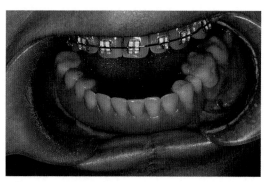

Fig. 43. Denture in place over Hader bar.

containing a floating shelf corresponding to the density of osteoprogenitor/stem cells (**Fig. 38**). The BMAC yielded 7.68×10^6 of CD44+ osteoprogenitor/stem cells, and cell adhesion molecules similar to those in PRP. The BMAC was added to the rhBMP-2/ACS sponges, which were cut into 1-cm squares and added to the CCFDAB to obtain a composite graft that satisfied the tissue engineering triangle (**Fig. 39**). The graft was

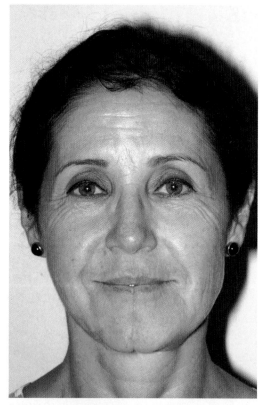

Fig. 44. The rhBMP-2/ACS-CCFDAB-BMAC graft achieved normal mandibular height and contour and improved facial contours.

placed and filled the defect, supported by a titanium plate and mesh for stability (**Fig. 40**).

The graft matured over 6 months into a solid ossicle of ideal bone height (**Fig. 41**) and mandibular contour into which five implants were placed (**Fig. 42**). These implants were allowed to osseointegrate for 6 months and were able to support a prosthesis (**Fig. 43**), and produced a marked improvement in facial contours (**Fig. 44**).

REFERENCES

1. Centers for Disease Control and Prevention. Total tooth loss among persons aged > or = 65 years. Selected states, 1995–1997. MMWR Morb Mortal Wkly Rep 1999;48(10):206–10.
2. Gift HC, Redford M. Oral health and quality of life. Clin Geriatr Med 1992;8:673–83.
3. Hollister MC, Weintraub JA. The association of oral status with systemic health, quality of life, and economic productivity. J Dent Educ 1993;57(12):901–12.
4. Reisine S, Locker D. Social, psychological, and economic impacts of oral conditions and treatments. In: Cohen LK, Gift HC, editors. Disease prevention and oral health promotion: socio-dental sciences in action. Copenhagen (Denmark): Munksgaard and la Federation Dentaire Internationale; 1995. p. 33–71.
5. Weintraub JA, Burt BA. Oral health status in the United States: tooth loss and edentulism. J Dent Educ 1985;49:368–78.
6. The Third National Health and Nutrition Examination Survey (NHANES III) 1988–1994, National Center for Health Statistics, Centers for Disease Control and Prevention, and the 1999 Behavioral Risk Factor Surveillance System (BRFSS), Centers for Disease Control and Prevention. Available at: http://drc.hhs.gov/report/dqs_tables/pdf/Table4_1_1.pdf. Accessed February 7, 2011.
7. Data sources: 1998 National Health Interview Survey, National Center for Health Statistics, Centers for Disease Control and Prevention and 1999 Behavioral Risk Factor Surveillance System, Centers for Disease Control and Prevention. Available at: http://drc.hhs.gov/report/dqs_tables/pdf/Table4_3_1.pdf. Accessed February 7, 2011.
8. Kim K, Lee CH, Kim BK, et al. Anatomically shaped tooth and periodontal regeneration by cell homing. J Dent Res 2010;89(8):842–7.
9. Jensen SS, Bosshardt DD, Buser D. Bone grafts and bone substitute materials. In: Buser D, editor. 20 Years of guided bone regeneration in implant dentistry. Chicago: Quintessence Publishing; 2009. p. 1–96.
10. Brånemark PI. Osseointegration and its experimental studies. J Prosthet Dent 1983;50:399–410.
11. Worthington P. History, development, and current status of osseointegration as revealed by experience in craniomaxillofacial surgery. In: Brånemark PI, Rydevik BL, Skalak R, editors. Osseointegration in skeletal reconstruction and joint replacement. Carol Stream (IL): Quintessence Publishing Co; 1997. p. 25–44.
12. Brånemark PI. Vital microscopy of bone marrow in rabbit. Scand J Clin Lab Invest 1959;11(Suppl 38):1–82.
13. Skalak R. Overview of previous development and biomechanics of osseointegration. In: Rydevik B, Brånemark PI, Skalak R, editors. International workshop on osseointegration in skeletal reconstruction and joint replacement. Göteborg (Sweden): The Institute for Applied Biotechnology; 1991. p. 45–56.
14. Sundgren JE, Bodö P, Lundström I. Auger electronspectroscopic of the interface between human tissue and implants of titaniumand stainless steel. J Colloid Interface Sci 1986;110:9–20.

15. Bjursten LM. The bone-implant interface in osseointegration. In: Rydevik B, Brånemark PI, Skalak R, editors. International workshop on osseointegration in skeletal reconstruction and joint replacement. Göteborg (Sweden): The Institute for Applied Biotechnology; 1991. p. 25–31.

16. Martin JY, Schwartz Z, Hummert TW, et al. Effect of titanium surface roughness on proliferation, differentiation, and protein synthesis of human osteoblast-like cells (MG63). J Biomed Mater Res 1995;29:389–401.

17. Lincks J, Boyan BD, Blanchard CR, et al. Response of MG63 osteoblast-like cells to titanium and titanium alloy is dependent on surface roughness and composition. Biomaterials 1998;19:2219–32.

18. Davies J, Hosseini MM. Histodynamics of endosseous wound healing. In: Davies JE, editor. Bone engineering. Toronto (Ontario): Em squared; 2000. p. 1.

19. Osborn JF, Newesely H. Dynamic aspects of the implant–bone interface. In: Heimke G, editor. Dental implants: materials and systems. München (Germany): Carl Hanser Verlag; 1980. p. 111.

20. Park JY, Davies JE. Red blood cell and platelet interactions with titanium implant surfaces. Clin Oral Implants Res 2000;11:530.

21. Park J, Gemmell CH, Davies JE. Platelet interactions with titanium: modulation of platelet activity by surface topography. Biomaterials 2001;19:2671.

22. Glowacki J, Rey C, Glimcher MJ, et al. A role of osteocalcin in osteoclast differentiation. J Cell Biochem 1991;45:1.

23. Masuda T, Salvi GE, Offenbacher S, et al. Cell and matrix reactions at titanium implants in surgically prepared rat tibiae. Int J Oral Maxillofac Implants 1997; 12:472.

24. Berton G, Lowell CA. Integrin signalling in neutrophils and macrophages. Cell Signal 1999;11:621.

25. McKee MD, Nanci A. Secretion of osteopontin by macrophages and its accumulation at tissue surfaces during wound healing in mineralized tissues: a potential requirement for macrophage adhesion and phagocytosis. Anat Rec 1996;245: 394.

26. Champagne CM, Takebe J, Offenbacher S, et al. Macrophage cell lines produce osteoinductive signals that include bone morphogenetic protein-2. Bone 2002; 30:26.

27. Wozney JM. The bone morphogenetic protein family and osteogenesis. Mol Reprod Dev 1992;32:160–7.

28. Wozney JM. Bone morphogenetic proteins. Prog Growth Factor Res 1989;1: 267–80.

29. Wozney JM. The bone morphogenetic protein family: multifunctional cellular regulators in the embryo and adult. Eur J Oral Sci 1998;106(Suppl 1):160–6.

30. Wozney JM, Rosen V, Byrne M, et al. Growth factors influencing bone development. J Cell Sci Suppl 1990;13:149–56.

31. Schaub RG, Wozney J. Novel agents that promote bone regeneration. Curr Opin Biotechnol 1991;2:868–71.

32. Zhou H, Hammonds R Jr, Findlay DM, et al. Differential effects of transforming growth factor-beta 1 and bone morphogenetic protein 4 on gene expression and differentiated function of preosteoblasts. J Cell Physiol 1993;155:112–9.

33. Wang EA, Israel DI, Kelly S, et al. Bone morphogenetic protein-2 causes commitment and differentiation in C3H10T1/2 and 3T3 cells. Growth Factors 1993;9: 57–71.

34. Cunningham NS, Paralkar V, Reddi AH. Osteogenin and recombinant bone morphogenetic protein 2B are chemotactic for human monocytes and stimulate

transforming growth factor B1 mRNS expression. Proc Natl Acad Sci U S A 1992; 89:11740–4.

35. Chiu-Jou Wu, Hsein-Kun Lu. Smad signal pathway in BMP-2-induced osteogenesis a mini review. J Dent Sci 2008;3(1):13–21 [in Chinese].

36. Nakashima K, Zhou X, Kunkel G, et al. The novel zinc finger-containing transcription factor Osterix is required for osteoblast differentiation and bone formation. Cell 2002;108:17–29.

37. Deckers MM, van Bezooijen RL, van der Horst G, et al. Bone morphogenetic proteins stimulate angiogenesis through osteoblast-derived vascular endothelial growth factor A. Endocrinology 2002;143(4):1545–53.

38. Li G, Cui Y, McIlmurray L, et al. rhBMP-2, rhVEGF165, rhPTN and thrombin-related peptide, TP508 induce chemotaxis of human osteoblasts and microvascular endothelial cells. J Orthop Res 2005;23:680–5.

39. Fiedler J, Röderer G, Günther KP, et al. BMP-2, BMP-4, and PDGF-bb stimulate chemotactic migration of primary human mesenchymal progenitor cells. J Cell Biochem 2002;87:305–12.

40. Arnaout MA, Goodman SL, Xiong JP. Coming to grips with integrin binding to ligands. Curr Opin Cell Biol 2002;14:641–51.

41. Schneider GB, Zaharias R, Seabold D, et al. Differentiation of preosteoblasts is affected by implant surface microtopographies. J Biomed Mater Res A 2004; 69:462–8.

42. Rezania A, Healy KE. Integrin subunits responsible for adhesion of human osteoblast-like cells to biomimetic peptide surfaces. J Orthop Res 1999;17:615–23.

43. Boyne PJ, Lilly LC, Marx RE, et al. De novo bone induction by recombinant human bone morphogenetic protein-2 (rhBMP-2) in maxillary sinus floor augmentation. J Oral Maxillofac Surg 2005;63:1693.

44. Fiorellini JP, Howell TH, Cochran D, et al. Randomized study evaluating recombinant human bone morphogenetic protein-2 for extraction socket augmentation. J Periodontol 2005;76:605.

45. Triplett GR, Nevins M, Marx RE, et al. Pivotal randomized, parallel evaluation of recombinant human bone morphogenetic protein-2/absorbable collagen sponge and autogenous bone graft for maxillary sinus floor augmentation. J Oral Maxillofac Surg 2009;67:1947–60.

46. Spagnoli DB. The application of recombinant human bone morphogenetic protein on absorbable collagen sponge (rhBMP-2/ACS) to reconstruction of maxillofacial bone defects. In: Vukicevic S, Sampath KT, editors. Bone Morphogenetic proteins: from local to systemic therapeutics. Basel (Switzerland): Birkhauser; 2008. p. 43–70.

47. Li XJ, Boyne P, Lilly L, et al. Different osteogenic pathways between rhBMP-2/ACS and autogenous bone graft in 190 maxillary sinus floor augmentation surgeries. J Oral Maxillofac Surg 2007;65(9 Suppl 1):36.

Index

Note: Page numbers of article titles are in **boldface** type.

Dent Clin N Am 55 (2011) 909–915
doi:10.1016/S0011-8532(11)00131-5
0011-8532/11/$ – see front matter © 2011 Elsevier Inc. All rights reserved.

dental.theclinics.com

United States Postal Service
Statement of Ownership, Management, and Circulation
(All Periodicals Publications Except Requester Publications)

1. Publication Title
Dental Clinics of North America

2. Publication Number
5 6 6 - 4 8 0

3. Filing Date
9/16/10

4. Issue Frequency
Jan, Apr, Jul, Oct

5. Number of Issues Published Annually
4

6. Annual Subscription Price
$240.00

7. Complete Mailing Address of Known Office of Publication (Not printer) (Street, city, county, state, and ZIP+4®)

Elsevier Inc.
360 Park Avenue South
New York, NY 10010-1710

Contact Person
Stephen Bushing

Telephone (Include area code)
215-239-3688

8. Complete Mailing Address of Headquarters or General Business Office of Publisher (Not printer)

Elsevier Inc., 360 Park Avenue South, New York, NY 10010-1710

9. Full Names and Complete Mailing Addresses of Publisher, Editor, and Managing Editor (Do not leave blank)

Publisher (Name and complete mailing address)

Kim Murphy, Elsevier, Inc., 1600 John F. Kennedy Blvd. Suite 1800, Philadelphia, PA 19103-2899

Editor (Name and complete mailing address)

Donald Mumford, Elsevier, Inc., 1600 John F. Kennedy Blvd. Suite 1800, Philadelphia, PA 19103-2899

Managing Editor (Name and complete mailing address)

Sarah Barth, Elsevier, Inc., 1600 John F. Kennedy Blvd. Suite 1800, Philadelphia, PA 19103-2899

10. Owner (Do not leave blank. If the publication is owned by a corporation, give the name and address of the corporation immediately followed by the names and addresses of all stockholders owning or holding 1 percent or more of the total amount of stock. If not owned by a corporation, give the names and addresses of the individual owners. If owned by a partnership or other unincorporated firm, give its name and address as well as those of each individual owner. If the publication is published by a nonprofit organization, give its name and address.)

Full Name	Complete Mailing Address
Wholly owned subsidiary of	4520 East-West Highway
Reed/Elsevier, US holdings	Bethesda, MD 20814

11. Known Bondholders, Mortgagees, and Other Security Holders Owning or Holding 1 Percent or More of Total Amount of Bonds, Mortgages, or Other Securities. If none, check box ☐ None

Full Name	Complete Mailing Address
N/A	

12. Tax Status (For completion by nonprofit organizations authorized to mail at nonprofit rates) (Check one)
The purpose, function, and nonprofit status of this organization and the exempt status for federal income tax purposes:
☐ Has Not Changed During Preceding 12 Months
☐ Has Changed During Preceding 12 Months (Publisher must submit explanation of change with this statement)

PS Form **3526**, September 2007 (Page 1 of 3 (Instructions Page 3)) PSN 7530-01-000-9931 PRIVACY NOTICE: See our Privacy policy in www.usps.com

---

13. Publication Title
Dental Clinics of North America

14. Issue Date for Circulation Data Below
July 2011

15. Extent and Nature of Circulation		Average No. Copies Each Issue During Preceding 12 Months	No. Copies of Single Issue Published Nearest to Filing Date
a. Total Number of Copies (Net press run)		1459	1300
b. Paid Circulation (By Mail and Outside the Mail)	(1) Mailed Outside-County Paid Subscriptions Stated on PS Form 3541 (Include paid distribution above nominal rate, advertiser's proof copies, and exchange copies)	599	555
	(2) Mailed In-County Paid Subscriptions Stated on PS Form 3541 (Include paid distribution above nominal rate, advertiser's proof copies, and exchange copies)		
	(3) Paid Distribution Outside the Mails Including Sales Through Dealers and Carriers, Street Vendors, Counter Sales, and Other Paid Distribution Outside USPS®	275	313
	(4) Paid Distribution by Other Classes Mailed Through the USPS (e.g. First-Class Mail®)		
c. Total Paid Distribution (Sum of 15b (1), (2), (3), and (4))	▲	874	868
d. Free or Nominal Rate Distribution (By Mail and Outside the Mail)	(1) Free or Nominal Rate Outside-County Copies Included on PS Form 3541	58	60
	(2) Free or Nominal Rate In-County Copies Included on PS Form 3541		
	(3) Free or Nominal Rate Copies Mailed at Other Classes Through the USPS (e.g. First-Class Mail)		
	(4) Free or Nominal Rate Distribution Outside the Mail (Carriers or other means)		
e. Total Free or Nominal Rate Distribution (Sum of 15d (1), (2), (3) and (4))	▲	58	60
f. Total Distribution (Sum of 15c and 15e)	▲	932	928
g. Copies not Distributed (See instructions to publishers #4 (page #3))	▲	527	372
h. Total (Sum of 15f and g)	▲	1459	1300
i. Percent Paid (15c divided by 15f times 100)		93.78%	93.53%

16. Publication of Statement of Ownership
☐ If the publication is a general publication, publication of this statement is required. Will be printed in the **October 2011** issue of this publication. ☐ Publication not required

17. Signature and Title of Editor, Publisher, Business Manager, or Owner

Stephen R. Bushing — Inventory / Distribution Coordinator

Date September 16, 2011

I certify that all information furnished on this form is true and complete. I understand that anyone who furnishes false or misleading information on this form or who omits material or information requested on the form may be subject to criminal sanctions (including fines and imprisonment) and/or civil sanctions (including civil penalties).

PS Form 3526, September 2007 (Page 2 of 3)

Moving?

Make sure your subscription moves with you!

To notify us of your new address, find your **Clinics Account Number** (located on your mailing label above your name), and contact customer service at:

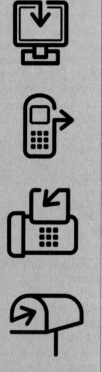

Email: journalscustomerservice-usa@elsevier.com

800-654-2452 (subscribers in the U.S. & Canada)
314-447-8871 (subscribers outside of the U.S. & Canada)

Fax number: 314-447-8029

Elsevier Health Sciences Division
Subscription Customer Service
3251 Riverport Lane
Maryland Heights, MO 63043